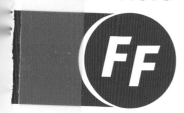

FAST FACTS

Indispensable Guides to Clinical Practice

Endometriosis

Second edition

Botros Rizk

Professor and Chief
Division of Reproductive Endocrinology and Infertility
Department of Obstetrics and Gynecology
University of South Alabama, Alabama, USA

Hossam Abdalla

Director of the Lister Fertility Clinic
The Lister Hospital, London, UK

D0191833

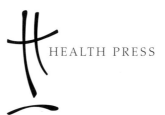

HEALTH PRESS

Oxford

Fast Facts – Endometriosis
First published 1998
Second edition September 2003

Text © 2003 Botros Rizk, Hossam Abdalla

© 2003 in this edition Health Press Limited
Health Press Limited, Elizabeth House, Queen Street, Abingdon, Oxford
OX14 3JR, UK
Tel: +44 (0)1235 523233
Fax: +44 (0)1235 523238

Fast Facts is a trademark of Health Press Limited

A CIP catalogue record for this title is available from the British Library.

ISBN 1-903734-35-5

Rizk, B (Botros)
Fast Facts – Endometriosis/
Botros Rizk, Hossam Abdalla

Medical illustrations by Dee McLean and Jane Fallows, London, UK.

Typesetting and page layout by Zed, Oxford, UK.

Printed by Fine Print (Services) Ltd, Oxford, UK.

Printed with vegetable inks on fully biodegradable and
recyclable paper manufactured from sustainable forests.

444 001
Low emissions
during production

Low
chlorine

Sustainable
forests

Glossary

adhesiolysis: separation/removal of adhesions

adnexal masses: enlarged parts of the Fallopian tubes or ovaries

AFS: American Fertility Society, now known as the ASRM

amenorrhea: absence of menstruation

anovulation: lack of ovulation

ASRM: American Society for Reproductive Medicine

blastocyst stage: stage at which an embryo implants in the uterus

blebs: blister-like lumps filled with fluid

catechol estrogens: hormones derived from amino acids

cervical atresia: closure of the neck of the womb

COH: controlled ovarian hyperstimulation

dyschezia: painful defecation

dysmenorrhea: pain before and during menstruation

dyspareunia: painful sexual intercourse

dysuria: pain on passing urine

endometrial atrophy: pseudopregnancy

endometrioma: tumor of abnormally placed endometrium

estradiol: natural estrogen used to control menopausal symptoms

fecundity rate: fertility ability rating

FSH: follicle-stimulating hormone

GIFT: gamete intrafallopian transfer

glandular epithelia: outer cell layer of glands

GnRH: gonadotropin-releasing hormone

GnRH analogs: drugs which initially superstimulate the pituitary gland to make more GnRH and then shut down GnRH production

GnRH antagonists: drugs which stop the production of GnRH

hematuria: blood in the urine

hirsutism: excessive growth of hair on face and body

humoral immune response: antibody response

hypermenorrhea: heavy menstrual bleeding

hyperplasia: abnormal growth in number of tissue cells, increasing the size of the organ

hyperprolactinemia: abnormally high production of the hormone prolactin

ICSI: intracytoplasmic sperm injection

implantation: penetration of and attachment to lining of womb by fertilized ovum

IUI: intrauterine insemination

IVF: in-vitro fertilization

LH: luteinizing hormone

lysis: destruction of living cells through rupture of membranes

macrophages: scavenging cells of the immune system

mesothelium: lining cells of the peritoneum, pleura and other body parts

metaplasia: abnormal change in tissue as a result of change in cells

occlusion: closing of an opening, or obstruction of a hollow part

oligomenorrhea: abnormally infrequent periods

oophorectomy: surgical removal of ovaries

parenchyma: the functional tissue of an organ

pathognomonic: uniquely characteristic of a disease

periovarian adhesions: adhesions around the ovaries

peritoneal fluid: lubricant secreted by the peritoneum

phagocytosis: destruction of foreign bodies by phagocytes

prostaglandins: hormone-like substances involved in many body processes (e.g. influencing blood clotting, inducing abortion, causing muscle contraction)

retrograde menstruation: retention of menstrual blood in the body

serum immunoassays: method of testing concentration of antibodies

sperm motility: 'swimming' action of sperm in seminal fluid

stroma: the tissue forming the supporting framework of an organ

superovulation: production of more than one or two eggs (ova) at one time

synthetic progestogens: drugs chemically and pharmacologically similar to natural hormone progesterone

uterine fibroids: benign tumors growing in the uterus wall

VEGF: vascular endothelial growth factor

Introduction

Endometriosis, the presence of tissue histologically similar to endometrium outside the uterine cavity and the myometrium, is one of the most common gynecologic conditions in women of reproductive age, but it remains one of the most complicated and baffling. It is estimated that over 5 million women in the USA have endometriosis, and it is thought to affect 10–25% of all women attending gynecologic clinics in the USA and the UK. Sufferers make up a sizeable proportion of those attending gynecologic practices, whether seeking help for infertility or because the condition has become chronic with disabling effects. Although it is not easy to determine how prevalent the disease is among the general population (at present, it can only be confirmed by laparoscopy or laparotomy), there are indications that it is increasing. One factor in this could be the considerable delay between the onset of pain and the surgical diagnosis – in the UK it is 8 years, in the USA it is about 10 years.

In addition to the physical effects of the disease, the psychological impact of endometriosis is also a cause for concern. Every practicing primary care provider and gynecologist should be aware of the feelings of frustration and consequent depression experienced by women with endometriosis.

On numerous occasions women have been referred to psychiatrists as 'mental cases', a 'psychologizing' of endometriosis that represents the failure of gynecologists to diagnose the condition. In one clinic, out of 850 laparoscopies performed in patients with pain of 6 months' duration or longer, histologically proven endometriosis or adhesions were found in 92%. After this treatment, their psychological profiles returned to near-normal, because when endometriosis was removed, pelvic pain improved.

We must stop the psychologizing of endometriosis. Gynecologists must not allow frustrated or ill-informed colleagues to dismiss patients as 'cranks' rather than diagnose and treat them or refer them to specialists who can do so.

Though the disease has been known for more than a century, it remains a challenge to gynecologists and primary care physicians. *Fast Facts – Endometriosis* presents healthcare professionals with the latest information to enable the patient to be treated with consideration and speed.

Epidemiology

The incidence of endometriosis remains unknown, because the disease is usually recorded as part of another investigation, for example into infertility or chronic pain in the abdomen or pelvis, or during another procedure such as sterilization. Many factors could account for the variations in the estimates of prevalence of endometriosis drawn from different investigations.

Prevalence of endometriosis

On the basis of hospital and surgical records. In the USA in 1980, among women aged 15–44 years, 6.3% of first diagnosis and 6.9% of all diagnoses for genitourinary problems were linked to endometriosis (National Center for Health Statistics). Between 1988 and 1990 the US National Hospital Discharge Survey, covering over 5 million gynecologic diagnoses, put endometriosis as first diagnosis at 11.2%. US Army records (1980–85) show that endometriosis was diagnosed in 6.2% of women undergoing gynecologic surgery. Another review from Houston, Texas, put the prevalence of endometriosis at 10.3%.

Smaller surgical case reports show a range of findings: when laparoscopy was performed for pelvic pain, a prevalence rate of 4–80% was reported for endometriosis compared with 2–80% for infertility. Endometriosis was reported in 4% of over 10 000 women undergoing tubal ligation.

In the UK, endometriosis was noted in 21% of women being investigated for infertility and in 6% being sterilized. For those with chronic abdominal pain, the incidence of endometriosis was 15%; among those having abdominal hysterectomy it was 25%.

On the basis of population studies. In the UK and the USA, three general epidemiological studies of endometriosis have been reported. In the UK, the Oxford Family Planning Association studied a cohort of 17 032 British women between 1968 and 1974. The authors reviewed the women's medical records up until the end of 1990 for a diagnosis of endometriosis at laparoscopy or laparotomy, identifying 142 in which endometriosis was the first diagnosis. One limitation of this study is that controls did not undergo laparoscopy and therefore some could have undiagnosed endometriosis.

Houston and co-authors reviewed the medical records of white residents of Rochester, Minnesota, USA, from 1970 to 1979, to find newly diagnosed cases of endometriosis. They had four diagnostic groups:

- histologically confirmed disease
- visualization of disease during surgery
- clinically probable diagnosis based on pain and positive examination
- clinically possible diagnosis based on examination alone.

From these data, the authors concluded a prevalence of between 2.5% and 3.3% – assuming that the endometriosis had an average duration of 10 years. However, should the duration be 25 years, the prevalence rate would be 6.2–8.2%. As there is known to be considerable delay in the diagnosis between the onset of pain symptoms and the surgical confirmation, prevalence rates should take this into account.

Kjerulff and colleagues used the self-reporting method (US Health Interview Survey, 1984–92), asking a random sample aged 18–50 years about their gynecologic problems of the previous year. Of 341 617 women surveyed, 211 had been diagnosed with endometriosis and 1666 reported having menstrual disorders. The authors acknowledged that the reported prevalence rates of 6.9/1000 for endometriosis and 53/1000 for menstrual disorders could be underestimates because many respondents were embarrassed to answer personal questions. Others had not reported their symptoms to a physician; some had forgotten about them.

Changes in prevalence. The available data show that gynecologic surgery for endometriosis has been on the rise. In 1965, approximately 130 000 hysterectomies were performed for endometriosis in the USA, compared with 390 000 in 1984 (the proportions are shown in Figure 1.1). Although the general trend was to an increase in the number of hysterectomies performed during this period (Figure 1.2), the proportion carried out for endometriosis rose from 9% to 19%, an

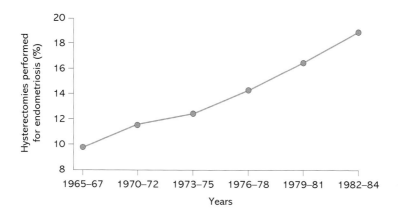

Figure 1.1 Proportion of hysterectomies performed in the USA for endometriosis. Source: US National Center for Health Statistics, Hyattsville, MD 1987.

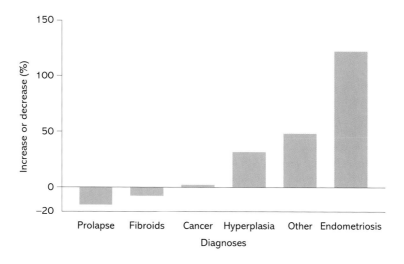

Figure 1.2 Changes in the indications for hysterectomy in the USA between 1965 and 1984. Source: Nezhat et al. 1995.

increase of 120%, which is unmatched by any other condition. It seems likely, given the dramatically increased frequency of surgical intervention for endometriosis, that the prevalence of the disease has increased.

Differences in characteristics of patients with endometriosis in the USA and the UK. An interesting investigation was undertaken by the Harvard Medical School in the US and the University of Oxford in the UK to study patient demographics in both countries. Only women with surgically diagnosed endometriosis were included (80 in the US and 187 in the UK). Most demographic characteristics were similar for the two groups, a finding supporting the universality of the disease process. However, patients in the US were diagnosed at a younger age than were patients in the UK, and more commonly presented with an ovarian mass. More UK women used oral contraceptives before diagnosis and were younger at first use. UK patients underwent fewer additional surgeries than US patients but reported that surgery alone provided the best relief of symptoms, whereas most US patients reported that surgical and medical therapy together provided the best relief of symptoms.

Risk factors. A number of factors appear to increase the risk of endometriosis (Table 1.1).

Race appears to be an important factor affecting susceptibility to endometriosis. The incidence of endometriosis is thought to be higher in Japanese women than in white women. Although some studies suggested that white women were more likely to develop endometriosis than black women, the difference was shown to be insignificant once confounding variables were taken into account.

Heredity. The heritable tendencies of endometriosis have long been recognized; the risk is 5% to 7% for first-degree relatives. This risk indicates that polygenic and multifactorial etiology is far more likely to be the cause than mendelian inheritance, as is the case for most adult-onset conditions in reproductive medicine (e.g. polycystic ovary disease and leiomyomata). In 1980, the first formal genetic study of endometriosis (by Simpson et al.) demonstrated that 5.9% of sisters and 8.1% of mothers of patients with endometriosis were affected. Of the patients' husbands' first-degree relatives (controls) only 1% had endometriosis. Women with an affected sibling or parent were more likely to have severe than mild or moderate endometriosis. Later studies have been consistent with these observations. In questionnaires from

TABLE 1.1

Factors affecting the risk of endometriosis

Increased risk

- Japanese origin
- Family history
- High estrogen status
- Age 30–44 years
- Increased menstrual flow and decreased cycle length
- Environmental factors, particularly dioxin exposure
- Increased peripheral body fat

Decreased risk

- Current and recent contraceptive users
- Current IUD users, possibly
- Smokers (possibly)

43 members of the Endometriosis Association reported by Lamb et al., endometriosis was present in 6.2% of mothers of probands and 3.8% of sisters, but in less than 1% of first-degree relatives of friends. In a Norwegian study of 515 cases, 3.9% of mothers and 4.8% of sisters of affected women had endometriosis, but only 0.7% of mothers and 0.6% of sisters of women who did not have endometriosis were affected. In the UK, a sixfold greater occurrence of endometriosis in first-degree relatives was noted. Higher concordance exists for monozygotic rather than dizygotic twins. Endometriosis as a cause of surgical menopause is more correlated in monozygotic than in dizygotic twins.

The search for genes predisposing individuals to endometriosis has traditionally been a choice between testing candidate genes for allelic association with endometriosis or conducting larger scale linkage studies to identify chromosomal regions by the affected sibling-pair method. The linkage approach using genome-wide scanning of informative polymorphic microsatellite markers to identify regions of significant excess sharing in affected siblings has been adopted by several groups in the UK, US and Australia. The International Endogene Study is a collaboration between the University of Oxford and the Australian Gene Cooperative Research Centre (CRC). This is the largest clinical resource for linkage and association studies in endometriosis. As of April 2002 the combined data set consists of more than 2500 families.

Hormonal. There is strong circumstantial evidence that endometriosis is dependent on steroid hormones. Traditionally, endometriosis was thought to be rare in premenarchal girls and postmenopausal women. However, there have been recent reports of endometriosis in premenarchal girls, and the Endometriosis Association Registry records occurrences in postmenopausal women.

Age. The commonest age for diagnosis is 25–44. However, it is possible that the age of onset of the disease is in the teen years and detection is delayed. A positive relationship between endometriosis and age has been observed, with a peak prevalence at 40 years of age. The risk of having endometriosis is increased among women aged 30–34 years ($r = 2.1$), 35–39 years ($r = 4.5$) and 40–44 years ($r = 6.1$) relative to women aged 25–29 years.

Environmental. Dioxins, polychlorinated dibenzo-*p*-dioxins and polychlorinated dibenzofurans are tricyclic aromatic hydrocarbons with a planar configuration. Tetrachlorodibenzo-*p*-dioxin (TCDD) is the prototype. Although contact with TCDD and dioxin-like substances can be occupational or accidental, they are generally encountered through eating foods in which dioxins have bioaccumulated in the food chain. Pesticides may contaminate grass which is eaten by cattle, for example, and then meat and dairy products from these animals are consumed by humans. Other sources of dioxins are natural events such as volcanic eruption or forest and wood-burning fires, and they are also encountered as byproducts of manufacturing (Table 1.2). The WHO currently recommends that the intake of TCCD should be no more than 10 pg/kg body mass/day.

Dioxins and endometriosis in rhesus monkeys. A direct relationship between dioxins and endometriosis in rhesus monkeys was

TABLE 1.2

Sources of dioxins

- Pesticides and herbicides
- Waste incineration
- Many types of metal production
- Fossil fuel and petrol refining
- Chlorine bleaching, for example in the manufacture of white paper

demonstrated by Rier et al. in a study in which animals exposed to dioxin (5–25 parts per trillion) over four years were found to have a much higher prevalence of endometriosis than controls. A direct dose-dependent relationship was shown.

Case control studies in humans. The relationship between endometriosis and dioxins has been investigated in several case-control studies. The cases and controls were drawn from populations with very low exposure in Israel, in Quebec and in Pennsylvania. All these studies are fairly small, and the results differ. Lebel et al. from Quebec reported no differences between cases and controls in serum levels of dioxin or dioxin-like chemicals. However, Mayani et al. from Israel reported that 8 out of 44 cases (18%) had blood samples positive for dioxin compared with 1 out of 35 (3%) of controls (OR = 7.6; 95% CI = 0.9, 170). Also, among the Stage III and IV (revised American Society for Reproductive Medicine classification, r-ASRM) cases, 25% (5 of 20 women) were positive for dioxin, whereas among Stage I and II cases 12.5% (3 of 24 women) were positive for dioxin.

Eskenazi et al. studied the frequency of endometriosis in a heavily exposed population. This population in Seveso, Italy, a town about 14 kilometers north of Milan, was exposed to high levels of TCDD as a result of an explosion which took place at a chemical plant on 10 July, 1976. This population has been exposed to the highest levels of TCDD known in humans; exposure was to relatively pure TCDD, and individual TCDD exposure could be measured from the blood which was collected and stored between 1976 and 1980. A doubled, non-significant, risk for endometriosis was found among women with serum

TCDD levels of 100 ppt or higher, but no clear dose–response relation. It would be interesting to know whether there is a threshold for that effect or a sub-population which may be particularly susceptible.

Evidence from molecular biology. Levels of cytochrome P450 gene products and other markers of the presence of dioxin were compared in endometriotic and eutopic endometrial tissues by molecular biological techniques. Levels of transcripts of the expression of the CYP1A1 gene, known to be induced by dioxin, were 8.7 times higher in endometriotic than in eutopic endometrial tissue. This increased expression may significantly increase P450 1A1 enzyme activity and thus promote the growth of endometriosis. It is postulated that the mechanism may involve the induction of formation of catechol estrogens, the activation of procarcinogens, or both.

Socioeconomic status. Only one of the studies examining the relationship between endometriosis and socioeconomic status has reported a positive association. The suggestion that endometriosis is a disease of white, middle-class, career-oriented, egocentric and perfectionist women has no scientific basis.

Menstrual and reproductive history. There is an association between endometriosis and certain menstrual patterns. The risk is greater in women who have:

- increased menstrual pain (Figure 1.3)
- increased duration of flow (Figure 1.3)
- decreased cycle length (Figure 1.3)
- uterine abnormalities which occlude normal menstrual flow
- had an early menarche.

These factors, together with the fact that women today have a greater number of menses than their Victorian counterparts, might partly explain the apparent increased incidence of the disease.

Generally, risk of endometriosis is decreased in women who have previously been pregnant. The longer the pregnancy, the greater the protective effect, though it appears to wane as the time since the last birth increases; a case control study showed the odds ratio for endometriosis was 4.5 in those who had not had a birth in 10 years relative to women of a similar age who had a delivery in the last

5 years.

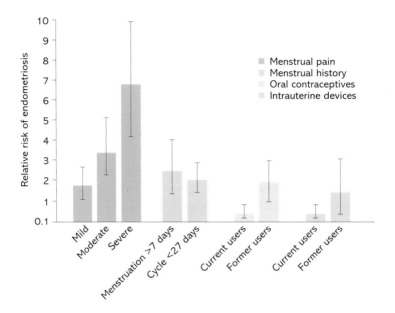

Figure 1.3 The risks of endometriosis related to menstrual pain, duration of menstrual flow and cycle length, oral contraceptive use ('former' here meaning 25–48 months previously), and use of intrauterine devices ('former' meaning 49–72 months previously).

Contraceptive use. In the only population-based cohort study conducted to date, Vessey and colleagues used the Oxford Family Planning Association study data to look for a relationship between contraceptive use and endometriosis (all cases were confirmed by laparoscopy). The authors reported that those currently or recently using oral contraceptives were less likely to have endometriosis than those who had never used oral contraceptives (Figure 1.3); there was no association between the disease and the duration of oral contraceptive use. It appears that oral contraceptives may mask endometriosis and its symptoms, which only emerge after oral contraceptives are discontinued.

In a study comparing women currently or recently using the intrauterine device (0–12 months) with former users (49–72 months), the risk was increased in the former users (Figure 1.3).

No association was found between diaphragm use and endometriosis.

Alcohol. Several of the gynecologic symptoms seen in women with endometriosis are also found in women who abuse alcohol or are dependent on it. Endometriosis patients have higher scores than the control patients on the Michigan Alcoholism Screening Test and consume more alcohol on a yearly basis.

The link between social and behavioral factors, alcohol and infertility were studied by Grodstein and co-workers: the odds ratio for endometriosis was 1.7 for moderate drinkers and 1.8 for heavy drinkers compared with infertile women who did not drink.

Caffeine. Grodstein looked at caffeine use in 1050 women with primary infertility and in 3833 women who had recently given birth. Those who drank more coffee were found to have a significant increase in risk of infertility as a result of tubal disease or endometriosis. This effect, however, seems more likely to be a result of the lifestyle of patients with endometriosis. Further epidemiological studies are required to evaluate these findings.

Smoking. Studies investigating the effects of smoking on reproductive function have produced conflicting results. Vessey et al. showed no association between endometriosis and smoking. Cramer, however, in a study of heavy smokers (> 1 pack of cigarettes/day) who had started to smoke before 17 years of age, showed an inverse relationship between endometriosis and smoking (odds ratio 0.5, 95% CI 0.3–0.9).

Smokers are relatively estrogen-deficient, as smoking appears to alter estrogen metabolism. They have an early natural menopause, a lower risk of endometrial cancer, an increased risk of osteoporotic fractures, and a reduced risk of uterine fibroids and benign breast disease. If high estrogen levels favor the development of endometriosis, as has been postulated, smokers may indeed be at lower risk.

However, smoking may account for a significant proportion of dioxin exposure. It has been estimated that someone smoking 1 pack/day takes in about 4.3 pg of polychlorinated dibenzodioxins/kg body weight/day.

Height, weight and body mass. In a study of body fat distribution (n = 176), after adjustment for age, body mass index, parity, age at menarche and intensity of menstrual flow, the risk of endometriosis was shown to be greater in women under 30 years of age with more peripheral body fat than those with more centralized fat. The lack of an effect in older women may be due to a progressive increase in waist circumference with age. This study was small and limited, but the authors' conclusion that greater peripheral body fat may be related to higher estrogen levels is consistent with the notion that endometriosis depends on estrogen.

Pathogenesis

Sir William Osler once said: 'He who knows endometriosis, knows gynecology'.

Endometriosis is defined as the presence of tissue histologically similar to endometrium outside the uterine cavity and the myometrium (Figure 1.4). Endometriosis externa is most commonly found in the pelvis (Figure 1.5), but may also occur in the abdominal cavity, the pleura and, very rarely, in the limbs and brain. A second variant, endometriosis interna, now called adenomyosis, is discussed in Chapter 10.

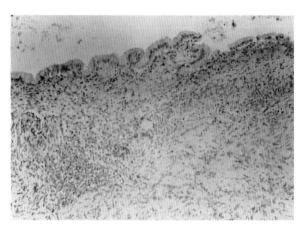

Figure 1.4 Biopsy of an endometrial cyst showing superficial endometrial tissue growing on the ovarian cortex. Reproduced with permission from Nezhat et al. 1995.

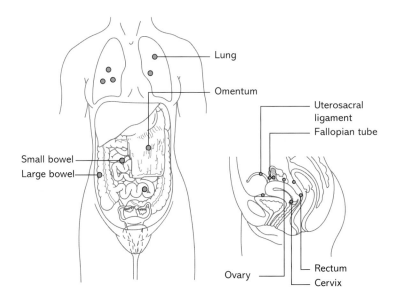

Figure 1.5 Sites of endometriosis: (a) non-pelvic and (b) pelvic.

Although the pathogenesis of endometriosis is complex and still incompletely understood, a number of theories have been developed (Table 1.3).

Implantation theory. The first description of the pathogenesis of endometriosis was made by von Rokitansky in 1860. Three essential conditions must be met in order to consider retrograde menstruation as the explanation for the pathogenesis of pelvic endometriosis:

- that retrograde menstruation occur and endometrial cells enter the peritoneal cavity through the fallopian tubes
- that menstrual blood contain viable endometrial cells that would adhere to the peritoneum with subsequent implantation and proliferation
- that the anatomical distribution of endometriosis in the pelvic cavity be correlated with the principles of transplantation for exfoliated cells.

Sampson's monumental work from Albany, New York, established the theory in the 1920s. He also described vascular dissemination and direct invasion. He suggested that blood from the uterine cavity at the

TABLE 1.3

Theories of pathogenesis

Implantation

- Retrograde menstruation
- Lymphatic dissemination
- Vascular dissemination
- Direct invasion
- Uterotubal

In situ

- Celomic metaplasia
- Müllerian duct remnants
- Wolffian duct remnants

Induction

- Endometrial-induced metaplasia

Combination

time of menstruation initiated endometriosis, and his observations were supported by several human and animal models.

Since retrograde menstruation occurs in at least 90% of all women, the question is why endometrial cells implant in only 10%. Is the endometrium of these women abnormal? It has been hypothesized that the presence of immunological defects in women with endometriosis leads to impaired clearance of the menstrual debris on the peritoneal surfaces. However, other investigators suggested that intrinsic molecular aberrations in the endometrium in women with endometriosis facilitate implantation of the endometrium on the pelvic peritoneum. These include deficient expression of an integrin and overexpression of complement 3 and certain cytokines. Furthermore, matrix metalloproteinase inhibitor type I is expressed in endometriosis but not in the endometrium. In women without endometriosis, there are no significant variations in vascular endothelial growth factor (VEGF) content in the eutopic glandular epithelium or stroma over the menstrual cycle. In patients with endometriosis, VEGF levels rise significantly in the eutopic glandular epithelium during the late secretory phase. This suggests that the endometrium of women with endometriosis is more likely to implant than that of women without endometriosis.

During the luteal phase, VEGF levels in both the glandular epithelium and stroma of red peritoneal endometriotic lesions are significantly higher than in black lesions, implying active angiogenesis in red lesions. The high levels of VEGF and the presence of matrix metalloproteinases (MMP-1) in red lesions throughout the cycle could be the key points of the implantation theory (Figure 1.6). Cells shed by such lesions under the influence of MMP-1 might implant elsewhere in the peritoneal cavity owing to the presence of VEGF.

In-situ development. If endometriosis does not occur as a result of retrograde menstruation, three theories propose that it develops in situ:
• celomic metaplasia theory
• müllerian duct remnant theory
• wolffian duct remnant theory.

Celomic metaplasia is an attractive theory that explains the occurrence of endometriosis at all sites, but evidence for it has yet to be established. If the peritoneal mesothelium has the potential to undergo metaplasia, this would be expected to occur in men too. While there are case reports in men, all involving the treatment of metastatic prostate cancer with high-dose estrogen, it is not celomic metaplasia. Furthermore, if endometriosis is to be attributed to celomic metaplasia, it should occur at sites where there are celomic membranes, such as the abdomen and thoracic cavities, but it is rare in the thorax. Finally, if it is similar to metaplasia elsewhere, it should occur with increasing frequency with advancing age. This is not the clinical pattern of endometriosis, as there is an abrupt halt when menstruation ceases at menopause. In postmenopausal women, the disease is associated with stimulation of pre-existing endometriosis by estrogen replacement therapy or endogenous estrogen production.

Müllerian duct remnant theory. This theory is based on the fact that rudimentary duplications of the müllerian system might be present in

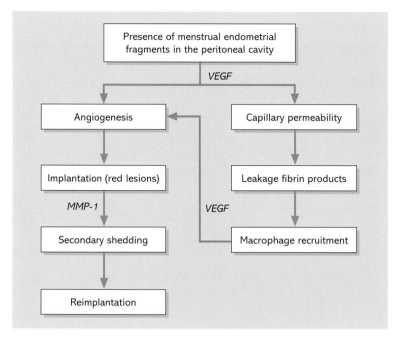

Figure 1.6 Hypothesis of the histogenesis of peritoneal endometriosis: the implantation theory.

areas adjacent to the müllerian ducts, allowing cells of müllerian origin to develop into functioning endometrium.

Wolffian duct remnant theory. This theory is similar to the müllerian duct remnant theory, but relates to the wolffian ducts.

Induction theory. The induction theory, introduced in 1955 by Levander and Normann, is based on the assumption that endometriosis results from differentiation of mesenchymal cells induced by substances released by degenerating endometrium that reach the peritoneal cavity. Other inductive influences, such as gonadal steroids and follicular fluid contents, have been postulated, and strong circumstantial evidence supports the dependence of endometriosis on steroid hormones.

Three different entities of endometriosis. Donnez and Nisolle suggested endometriosis is an organ-dependent disease. Peritoneal endometriosis, ovarian endometriosis, and adenomyotic nodules of the rectovaginal septum are three different entities. Peritoneal endometriosis occurs as a result of retrograde implantation, ovarian endometriosis as a result of celomic metaplasia, and rectovaginal endometriosis is a consequence of the remnants of the müllerian ducts.

Endometriosis and cancer. Tumors arising in endometriosis are predominantly of low grade and confined to the site of origin, and endometriotic lesions transform into malignancies in only approximately 0.7% to 1% of patients. Endometrioid cancer is the most frequent histological type (70%); there have also been cases of clear-cell carcinoma (14%). Atypical glandular changes have been found in 3.5% to 6% of cases of ovarian endometriosis. Malignant transformation involving the obliterated rectovaginal pouch has been reported with the use of opposed estrogen therapy, mestranol/norethynodrel or medroxyprogesterone acetate.

Ovarian carcinoma can cause cul-de-sac and uterosacral ligament nodularity and must therefore be investigated. Rapidly growing endometriomas and those larger than 10 cm should be sectioned carefully to search for malignant foci.

In an interesting article, Duczman and Ballweg noted that cancer and endometriosis share a number of similarities:
- abnormal growth of tissue with the ability to invade other tissues and organs
- reduced natural killer cell activity
- certain oncogenes in common
- angiogenesis
- loss of heterozygosity
- matrix metalloproteinases
- defective apoptosis.

The authors reviewed the relationship between endometriosis and cancer in four studies, which suggested that an elevated risk of breast cancer, ovarian cancer, non-Hodgkins lymphoma and melanoma exists in women with endometriosis. The Endometriosis Association study also indicates elevated risks of such cancers in the families of women with endometriosis.

Classification of endometriosis

Various attempts have been made to classify the different stages of endometriosis so that the outcome of treatments can be compared with a certain degree of accuracy. The system most widely used today has evolved from the classification originally developed in 1979 by the American Fertility Society (AFS), which is now known as the American Society for Reproductive Medicine (ASRM).

The ASRM classification (1996) provides a means of recording information about disease extent and morphology (Figure 1.7) along with the use of color photographs to ensure consistency in describing the disease appearance (endometriosis may have many different appearances). The extent of the disease is classified into stages I–IV according to the scoring system shown.

Appearance of endometriotic tissue.

Ovarian endometriotic cysts. This diagnosis should be confirmed by histology, or by the presence of four significant features:
- cyst diameter < 12 cm
- adhesions to pelvic side wall and/or broad ligament
- endometriosis on the surface of the ovary
- tarry thick brown ('chocolate') fluid content.

Cul-de-sac obliteration. For this to be complete, no peritoneum should be visible between the uterosacral ligaments.

Morphology of peritoneal and ovarian implants. These should be categorized as red (red, pink and clear lesions); white (white, yellow-brown and peritoneal defects), and black (black and blue lesions). The percentage of involvement of each implant type should be documented.

Stages of endometriotic tissue growth. Four different stages can be distinguished during the development of the disease (Figure 1.8). As the disease progresses, several stages can coexist at the same site (e.g. early active lesions can disappear or develop into fibrotic lesions).

Microscopic endometriosis. If the peritoneum appears to be normal macroscopically, an intraperitoneal lesion may be identified by scanning electron microscopy. This appears as areas of tall and ciliated epithelium, which noticeably replace the mesothelium. Another

Stage I (minimal)	1–5
Stage II (mild)	6–15
Stage III (moderate)	16–40
Stage IV (severe)	> 40

Total

	ENDOMETRIOSIS		< 1 cm	1–3 cm	> 3cm
PERITONEUM		Superficial	1	2	4
		Deep	2	4	6
OVARY	R	Superficial	1	2	4
		Deep	4	16	20
	L	Superficial	1	2	4
		Deep	4	16	20
	POSTERIOR CULDESAC OBLITERATION		Partial		Complete
			4		40
	ADHESIONS		< 1/3 Enclosure	1/3–2/3 Enclosure	> 2/3 Enclosure
OVARY	R	Filmy	1	2	4
		Dense	4	8	16
	L	Filmy	1	2	4
		Dense	4	8	16
TUBE	R	Filmy	1	2	4
		Dense	4*	8*	16
	L	Filmy	1	2	4
		Dense	4*	8*	16

*If the fimbriated end of the fallopian tube is completely enclosed, change the point assignment to 16.
Denote appearance of superficial implant types as red [(R) red, red-pink, flamelike, vesicular blobs, clear vesicles], white [(W) opacifications, peritoneal defects, yellow-brown], or black [(B) black, hemosiderin deposits, blue]. Denote percent of total described as R____%, W____% and B____%. Total should equal 100%.

Additional endometriosis: _____   Associated pathology: _____
_____   _____

To be used with normal
tubes and ovaries

To be used with abnormal
tubes and ovaries

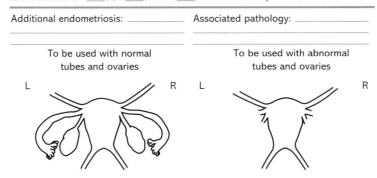

Figure 1.7 American Society for Reproductive Medicine revised classification of endometriosis.

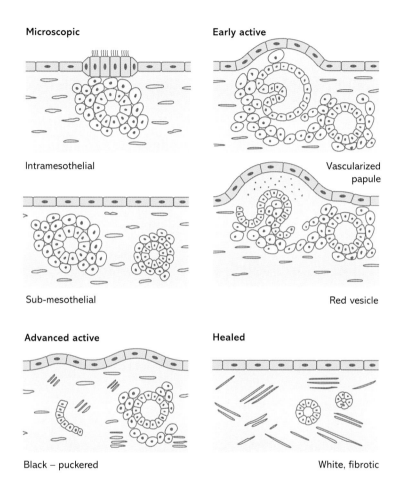

Microscopic

Intramesothelial

Sub-mesothelial

Early active

Vascularized papule

Red vesicle

Advanced active

Black – puckered

Healed

White, fibrotic

Figure 1.8 Evolution of peritoneal endometriosis.

microscopic appearance is the presence of endometrial glands and stroma under a normal mesothelium.

   Early active endometriosis. Polyps, vesicles and papules may be the earliest lesions seen and may appear to be either solid or fluid-filled. They are highly vascular and non-fibrotic. The glands are usually in a proliferative or secretory phase, not always in phase with the eutopic endometrium. Some lesions are very active in prostaglandin production.

Advanced active endometriosis. The typical pigmented hemorrhagic and fibrotic endometriotic deposits known as the classic lesions can be seen and are generally out of phase with the eutopic endometrium.

Healed endometriosis. White scarred lesions are indicative of healed endometriosis. Occasionally, calcified deposits can be seen and active glands can be found among fibrotic end-stage lesions.

Three-dimensional architecture of endometriosis. Donnez and colleagues applied advanced stereographic computer technology to identify two types of implants (Figure 1.9). In the first, composed of cylinder-like glands without ramifications, the glandular epithelia are regularly distributed in the stromal structure, which is also regular. The second type is composed of glands with ramifications; luminal structures are connected to each other, and finger-like epithelial structures appear to invade the stroma.

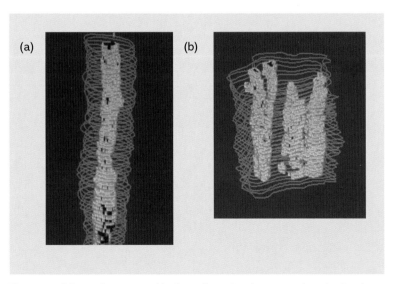

Figure 1.9 Advanced stereographic three-dimensional computer imaging has been used to identify two types of endometrial implant. (a) Regular distribution of the glandular epithelium in the stroma. (b) Glands with ramifications and interconnection of structures. Reproduced with permission from Nezhat et al. 1995.

Key points – Epidemiology and pathogenesis

- Prevalence estimates, based on hospital and population studies, suggest that endometriosis occurs in 7% of the female population, 4–80% of female patients with pelvic pain, and 2–80% of female patients undergoing laparoscopy for infertility.
- Over a 30-year period in the USA, hysterectomies for endometriosis have increased from 9% to 19% of all hysterectomies.
- Endometriosis has polygenic and multifactorial heritability; first-degree female relatives of women with endometriosis have an increased risk of developing this disease themselves.
- Environmental causes such as exposure to dioxins may be implicated in the development of endometriosis.
- There are several theories about pathogenesis; the most widely accepted is implantation from retrograde menstruation.
- There may be three types of endometriosis of different, organ-dependent etiologies: peritoneal, ovarian and rectovaginal.
- Like cancer, endometriosis involves tissue invasion, angiogenesis and defective apoptosis.

Key references

American Fertility Society: Revised classification of endometriosis. *Fertil Steril* 1985;43:351.

American Society for Reproductive Medicine. Revised American Society for Reproductive Medicine classification of endometriosis. *Fertil Steril* 1997;67:817.

Ballweg ML. Public testimony to the US Senate Committee on Labor and Human Resources, Subcommittee on Aging, May 5, 1993.

Berger GS. Endometriosis: How many women are affected? *Endometriosis Association Newsletter* 1993;14:4–6.

Berger GS. Epidemiology of endometriosis. In: Nezhat CR, Berger GS, Nezhat FR et al., eds. *Endometriosis: Advanced Management and Surgical Techniques.* New York: Springer, 1995:chapter 1, 3–17.

Boling RO, Abbasi R, Ackerman G et al. Disability from endometriosis in the United States Army. *J Reprod Med* 1988;33:49–52.

Bulun SE, Zeytoun KM, Kilick G. Expression of dioxin-related transactivating factors and target genes in human ectopic endometrial and endometriotic tissues. *Am J Obstet Gynecol 2000;182:767–75.*

Cramer DW, Wilson E, Stillman RJ et al. The relation of endometriosis to menstrual characteristics, smoking, and exercise. *JAMA* 1986;255: 1904–8.

Donnez J, Nisolle M. Endometriosis is an organ-dependent disease. Peritoneal endometriosis, ovarian endometriosis and adenomyotic nodules of the rectovaginal septum are three different entities. In: Lemay A, Maheux R, eds. *Understanding and Managing Endometriosis: Advances in Research and Practice.* New York: Parthenon, 1999:chapter 4, 17–29.

Duczman L, Ballweg ML. *Endometriosis and Cancer: What is the connection?* In: Ballweg ML. *Endometriosis: the Complete Reference for Taking Charge of Your Health.* New York: McGraw-Hill, 2004:chapter 8, 180–240.

Eskenazi B, Mocarelli P, Warner M et al. Serum dioxin concentrations and endometriosis: a cohort study in Seveso, Italy. *Environ Health Perspect* 2002;110:629–34.

Eskenazi B, Warner M. Epidemiology of endometriosis. *Endometriosis. Obstet Gynecol Clin N Am* 1997;24: 235–58.

Hadfield R, Mardon H, Barlow D, Kennedy S. Delay in the diagnosis of endometriosis: a survey of women from the USA and the UK. *Hum Reprod* 1996;11:878–80.

Halme J, Sahakian V. Endometriosis: pathophysiology and presentation. In: Keye WR, Chang RJ, Rebar RW et al., eds. *Infertility – evaluation and treatment.* Philadelphia: WB Saunders, 1995:496–508.

Houston EE, Noller KL, Melton J III, Selwyn BJ. The epidemiology of pelvic endometriosis. *Clin Obstet Gynecol* 1988;31:787–800.

Kjerulff KH, Erickson BA, Langenberg PW, Chronic gynecological conditions reported by US women: Findings from the National Health Information Survey, 1984 to 1992. *Am J Public Health* 1996;86:195.

Kuohung W, Jones GL, Vitonis BA et al. Characteristics of patients with endometriosis in the United States and the United Kingdom. *Fertil Steril* 2002;78:767–72.

Mahmood TA, Templeton A. Prevalence and genesis of endometriosis. *Hum Reprod* 1991;6: 544–9.

Mayani A, Barel S, Soback S, Almagor M. Dioxin concentrations in women with endometriosis. *Hum Reprod* 1997;12:373–5.

Moen MH, Magnus P. The familial risk of endometriosis. *Acta Obstet Gynecol Scand* 1993;72:560–4.

National Center for Health Statistics. Hysterectomies in the United States, 1965–84. Hyattsville, MD: National Center for Health Statistics, 1987; Vital and Health Statistics, Series 13, Data from the National Health Survey, No. 92, DHHS Pub No. (PHS) 88-1753.

Rier SE, Martin D, Bowman RE. Endometriosis in rhesus monkeys (*Macaca mulatta*) following chronic exposure to 2,3,7,8-tetrachlorodibenzo-*p*-dioxin. *Fundam Appl Toxicol* 1993;21: 433–41.Sampson JA. Peritoneal endometriosis due to menstrual dissemination of endometrial tissue into the peritoneal cavity. *Am J Obstet Gynecol* 1927;14:422–69.

Shaw RW, ed. *Advances in reproductive endocrinology: endometriosis*, vol 1. Carnforth, Lancs: Parthenon, 1990.

Simpson JL, Bischoff FZ, Kamat A et al. Genetics of endometriosis. *Endometriosis. Obstet Gynecol Clin N Am* 2003;30:21–40.

Simpson JL, Elias S, Malinak LR, Buttram VC Jr. Heritable aspects of endometriosis. I. Genetic studies. *Am J Obstet Gynecol* 1980;137:327–31.

Treloar S, Hadfield R, Montgomery G. The International Endogene Study: a collection of families for genetic research in endometriosis. *Fertil Steril* 2002;78:679–85.

Van der Linden PJQ. Theories on the pathogenesis of endometriosis. *Hum Reprod* 1996;11(suppl 3):53–65.

Vessey MP, Villard-Mackintosh L, Painter R. Epidemiology of endometriosis in women attending family planning clinics. *BMJ* 1993;306:182–4.

While it is easy to understand that advanced and severe endometriosis can cause disruption in the pelvis resulting in mechanical infertility, it is not similarly appreciated in general that minimal and mild endometriosis could have an impact on a woman's conceiving and achieving a live birth.

A controversial question: Does endometriosis cause infertility?

Evers and Dunselmen suggest that endometriosis is not a disease but an epiphenomenon. They elegantly discuss three issues related to a link between endometriosis and infertility, and conclude that there is insufficient evidence to support the contention that endometriosis per se causes infertility. They argue that endometriosis is not more frequent in subfertile women, that endometriosis patients do not have a lower fecundity rate, and that treatment does not improve pregnancy rate. On the first issue, they highlight the fact that 6–12% of random biopsies from normal peritoneum in patients without endometriosis do show endometriosis histologically. They hypothesize that if several biopsies per patient were performed instead of one, then the recorded incidence would be higher, and that if these biopsies were performed on 100% of the patients, then the incidence would increase further, to almost 100%. On the second issue, they suggested that the best way to determine the pregnancy rate in endometriosis without treatment is to compare the pregnancy rate in patients with untreated mild endometriosis with that in fertile normal women. However, this is not possible. Therefore, as a second-best, they compared the pregnancy rate in 2026 patients with unexplained infertility and in patients with endometriosis in the control group of the randomized controlled studies on endometriosis treatment. They found the pregnancy rates to be very similar (33% versus 28%). The rate in published studies of women with endometriosis undergoing artificial insemination by donor is comparable to that of women without laparoscopic evidence of endometriosis (64% versus 51%).

They also argued that the five randomized studies on medical therapy for endometriosis have shown no impact on the pregnancy rate whatsoever. They admitted that the only randomized surgical study, the Canadian Endometriosis Study, showed an improvement in pregnancy rate after the surgical treatment of mild and minimal endometriosis; however, the treatment effect was moderate.

On the other hand, many studies of operative laparoscopy suggest that the incidence of endometriosis in women undergoing tubal sterilization is very low compared with that in women undergoing evaluation of infertility. Some of the earlier studies of artificial insemination by donor of women with endometriosis suggest a lower pregnancy rate. Thus, while medical treatment apparently has no impact on the pregnancy outcome, there is more evidence that surgery improves the outcome. Therefore, this controversy will continue until more research can determine the links between endometriosis and infertility.

Factors associated with infertility

There are a number of possible mechanisms that can lead to infertility in patients with mild-to-moderate endometriosis (Table 2.1) or more severe endometriosis.

Peritoneal fluid abnormalities.

Increase in fluid volume. While several studies have shown an increase in the volume of peritoneal fluid in women with pelvic endometriosis, the correlation between fluid volumes and fertility outcome has not been similarly consistent.

Reduced sperm motility and binding. The peritoneal fluid from women with endometriosis has a negative impact on sperm motility, and sperm binding to the zona pellucida has been shown to be reduced in vitro.

Interleukins and tumor necrosis factor. Recent research has shown that interleukins (such as IL-1) and tumor necrosis factor alpha (TNF-α) in the peritoneal fluid of endometriosis patients are involved in inhibiting sperm motility and function, oocyte fertilization, and embryo growth.

TABLE 2.1

Possible mechanisms of infertility in patients with mild-to-moderate endometriosis

Changes in peritoneal fluid

- Increase in volume
- Reduced sperm motility and binding
- Presence of interleukins and tumor necrosis factor
- Increased prostaglandin levels
- Increased number of macrophages

Eutopic endometrium abnormalities

Myometrial and peristalsis abnormalities

Follicular environment and embryo quality

- Increased progesterone and interleukin-6
- Decreased vascular endothelial growth factor

Ovulation disorders

- Anovulation
- Hyperprolactinemia
- Abnormal follicular genesis
- Premature follicular rupture
- Luteinized unruptured follicles
- Luteal phase defect

Pelvic pain

Immunological abnormalities

- T-lymphocytes
- Antigen-specific B-lymphocyte activation
- Non-specific B-lymphocyte activation
- Antiendometrial antibodies

Spontaneous abortion

Implantation disorders

Prostaglandin levels. Increased prostaglandin levels in the peritoneal fluid of patients with endometriosis is another possible explanation of infertility. Prostaglandins alter tubal motility and collection of oocytes, and can lead to luteinized unruptured follicle syndrome and defects in the corpus luteum.

Macrophages. The number of macrophages in the peritoneal fluid is increased in women with pelvic endometriosis. The increase is associated with increased production of superoxides and oxygen free radicals, and thus with reduced sperm motility.

Eutopic endometrium abnormalities. The biochemical abnormalities in the eutopic endometrium of women with endometriosis are increasingly well defined and include altered local immune cell population, aberrant expression of proinflammatory chemotactic cytokines, impaired expression of differentiation markers and altered local steroid biosynthesis and metabolism.

Myometrial architecture and peristalsis abnormalities. Structural abnormalities of the uterine wall in women with endometriosis and infertility have been visualized by transvaginal sonography and magnetic resonance imaging. It has been suggested that uterine hyperperistalsis and dysperistalsis cause dysfunctions of the mechanism of rapid sperm transport in patients with endometriosis and infertility.

Follicular environment and embryo quality. Analyses of IVF and oocyte donation programs have suggested that the quality of the oocytes and embryos is impaired in patients with endometriosis. Pellicer et al. investigated the endocrine, paracrine and autocrine conditions during folliculogenesis in women with and without endometriosis. They found that changes in steroid synthesis during folliculogenesis, and in cytokine release by ovarian and blood cells, may result in oocytes and embryos of lower quality, and thus in infertility in patients with endometriosis. Further studies showed that the embryos have a reduced ability to implant.

Ovulation disorders in vivo.

Anovulation has been reported in 17–27% of patients with endometriosis. In some cases, combining treatment of the disease with induction of ovulation appears to increase the pregnancy rate.

Hyperprolactinemia has been reported in several studies of patients with different stages of endometriosis. It seems, however, that the conditions coexist and there is insufficient evidence to demonstrate a causal relationship.

Abnormal follicular dynamics have been reported, namely abnormal rates of follicular development and premature follicular rupture.

Luteal phase defect (LPD), detected by out-of-phase endometrial development or asynchronous development of endometrial glands and stroma, could be the consequence of abnormal follicular development, inadequate production of progesterone or lack of response of the endometrium to progesterone.

Luteinized unruptured follicle syndrome has been described in monkeys with surgically induced periovarian endometriotic adhesions. Theoretically, a decrease in luteinizing hormone (LH) receptors could be the underlying mechanism, but ultrasound studies have failed to show a consistent increase in incidence of this syndrome in patients with endometriosis.

Pelvic pain. Pain can lead to a reduction in the frequency of intercourse and, therefore, reduce the likelihood of pregnancy.

Immunological abnormalities.

T-lymphocytes. As endometriosis involves transplantation of autologous endometrium, and T-lymphocytes are concerned with the rejection of homografts, changes in T-lymphocyte function have long been suspected. Controversy exists, however, regarding the pattern of circulating leukocytes, as some, but not all, investigators have reported decreased numbers of lymphocytes. To add confusion, increased numbers of T-cells and of B-cells and higher CD4:CD8 ratios in blood and peritoneal fluid have also been reported.

Some researchers suggest that a subset of T-lymphocytes is functionally deficient in women with endometriosis. Recently, a specific deficiency in lymphocyte-mediated cytotoxicity towards autologous endometrial cells was observed and thought to be caused by dysfunction of natural killer (NK) lymphocytes. The lower cytotoxic effect has been confirmed by other investigators, but not NK cell dysfunction. A definitive mechanism by which altered T-cell function could cause infertility has not yet emerged.

B-lymphocytes. An autoimmune syndrome characterized by polyclonal B-lymphocyte activation has been suggested as a cause for infertility, though the exact mechanism is unclear.

Antiendometrial antibodies. Antibodies directed towards endometrial cell antigens have been reported in the serum of women with endometriosis, but the reason for their existence is controversial. Antiendometrial antibodies have also been detected in women with a wide range of pelvic pathologies.

Spontaneous abortion. An increased incidence of spontaneous abortion has been reported in patients with endometriosis, with a corresponding decrease after endometriosis has been treated. Abnormalities in prostaglandin function could be the mechanism. In a non-randomized study of patients with endometriosis, two-thirds of whom had suffered a previous miscarriage, the pregnancy rate was similar whether these patients had corrective surgery or not, but the miscarriage rate was higher in the group which had not been treated.

Implantation. Integrins are essential for cell adhesion. A deficiency of integrin $\alpha_3\beta_v$, a component of the embryo implantation cascade in the uterus, may reduce the likelihood of embryo implantation in women with early-stage endometriosis. However, this can apparently be corrected when the disease is treated. This interesting theory awaits further investigation and clinical studies.

Mechanical pelvic factors. Pelvic endometriosis can cause significant adhesions with distortion of the architecture. This interferes with both the release of the oocytes and their transfer into the fallopian tubes (Figure 2.1 and Table 2.2).

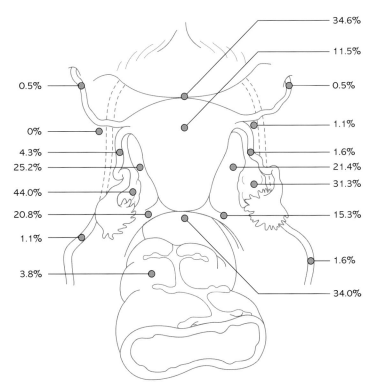

34.6%

11.5%

0.5%

0%

4.3%

25.2%

44.0%

20.8%

1.1%

3.8%

0.5%

1.1%

1.6%

21.4%

31.3%

15.3%

1.6%

34.0%

Figure 2.1 Distribution of endometriotic implants found at laparoscopy in 182 infertility patients. The numbers represent the proportion of all patients with implants at that site. Data from Jenkins S, Olive DL, Haney AF. *Obstet Gynecol* 1986;67:335–8.

TABLE 2.2

Pelvic factors and infertility in patients with moderate-to-severe endometriosis

- Adhesions with distortion of pelvic architecture interfering with the release of the oocytes and the tubal pick-up of these oocytes
- Fimbrial distortion or even occlusion can occur
- Hydrosalpinx can occur if the distal end of the tube is damaged
- Tubal narrowing and constriction
- Proximal tubal obstruction

Key points – Endometriosis and infertility

- The relationship between advanced endometriosis and infertility is clear. In minimal and mild disease, however, it remains controversial .
- Severe endometriosis can result in infertility by causing adhesions, fimbrial distortion, phimosis, occlusion, hydrosalpinx and proximal tubal obstruction.
- Mild and moderate endometriosis may cause infertility by causing peritoneal abnormalities, ovulatory dysfunction or immunologic defects.
- Ovulatory disorders in endometriosis include anovulation, abnormal follicular dynamics, luteal phase defect and luteinized unruptured follicle syndrome.
- In-vitro fertilization and oocyte donation studies suggest that endometriosis affects fertility by reducing the quality of oocytes rather than implantation.

Key references

Badawy SZ, Cuenca V, Marshall L et al. Cellular components in peritoneal fluid in infertile patients with and without endometriosis. *Fertil Steril* 1984;42:704–8.

Dheenadayalu K, Mak I, Gordts S. Aromatase P450 messenger RNA expression in eutopic endometrium is not a specific marker for pelvic endometriosis. *Fertil Steril* 2002; 78:825–35.

Evers JL, Dunselman GAJ. Endometriosis is not a disease but an epiphenomenon. In: Lemay A, Maheux R, eds. *Understanding and Managing Endometriosis: Advances in Research and Practice*. New York: Parthenon, 1999:chapter 5, 31–40.

Grunert GM, Franklin RR. Pathogenesis of infertility in endometriosis. In: Nezhat CR, Berger GS, Nezhat FR et al., eds. *Endometriosis: Advanced Management and Surgical Techniques*. New York: Springer, 1995:chapter 6, 45–59.

Hill JA. Immunology and Endometriosis: Fact, Artifact, or Epiphenomenon? *Endometriosis. Obstet Gynecol Clin N Am* 1997;24:291–306.

Jenkins S, Olive DL, Haney AF. Endometriosis. Pathogenetic implications of the anatomic distribution. *Obstet Gynecol* 1986;67:335.

Oosterlynck DF, Cornille FJ, Waer M et al. Women with endometriosis show a defect in natural killer activity resulting in a decreased cytotoxicity to autologous endometrium. *Fertil Steril* 1991;56:45–51.

Pellicer A, Albert C, Garrido N et al. The pathophysiology of endometriosis-associated infertility: follicular environment and embryo quality. *J Reprod Fertil* 2000;55(suppl):109–19.

Prough SG, Aksel S, Gilmore SM et al. Peritoneal fluid fractions from patients with endometriosis do not promote two-cell mouse embryo growth. *Fertil Steril* 1990;54:927–30.

Rizk B, Aboulghar M, Smitz J et al. The role of vascular endothelial growth factor and interleukins in the pathogenesis of severe ovarian hyperstimulation syndrome. *Hum Reprod Update* 1997;3:255–66.

Zreik TG, Olive DL. Pathophysiology: The biologic principles of disease. Endometriosis. *Obstet Gynecol Clin N Am* 1997;24:259–68.

An accurate clinical assessment is essential to identify those women most at risk and those who require further evaluation (Table 3.1). Correct diagnosis will prevent unnecessary treatments, debilitating chronic pain and, perhaps, in younger sufferers, infertility.

Endometriosis is almost always detected in women of reproductive age, most commonly between 25 and 29 years. The disease may also be found in early adolescents, especially those with partial or complete obstruction due to müllerian anomalies, such as cervical atresia or obstructed rudimentary uterine horns. Endometriosis is also reported in postmenopausal women, according to the Endometriosis Association Registry in the USA.

It is important to take a detailed history to identify the presence of any risk factors, and it is essential to ask about the family history, because of growing evidence suggesting a genetic component to the disease. Members of the same family may also share similar environmental conditions. In patients with a family link to the disease, endometriosis tends to be at a more advanced stage and behaves in a more aggressive fashion at presentation.

Symptoms and signs

The most common symptoms of endometriosis are dysmenorrhea and chronic pelvic pain unrelieved by analgesics (Table 3.2). Over half of affected patients complain of unilateral or bilateral pain typically beginning 1–2 days before menstruation and lasting throughout the flow. Rectal pressure and low back ache are also common symptoms.

The severity of the pain does not correlate with the stage of the disease. Patients with minimal or mild endometriosis may have active disease and significant symptoms, while patients with severe endometriosis could be completely pain-free. Over 50% of women with both pelvic pain and dysmenorrhea are found to have endometriosis at laparoscopy.

TABLE 3.1

Diagnosis of endometriosis

History

- Patient of reproductive age
- Short menstrual cycle (< 27 days)
- Partial or complete obstruction due to müllerian anomalies
- Infertility or long gap since last pregnancy
- Family history of endometriosis
- Patient with history of asthma, allergy or eczema

Symptoms and signs

- Dysmenorrhea
- Chronic pelvic pain
- Infertility
- Dyspareunia
- Premenstrual spotting
- Menstrual irregularities
- Low back pain
- Gastrointestinal complaints
- Dyschezia

Physical findings

- Nodules along the uterosacral ligaments
- Adnexal masses due to endometriomas (e.g. ovarian cysts)
- Fixed retroversion of the uterus

Investigations

- Laparoscopy (the most useful diagnostic tool)
- Microlaparoscopy (minimally invasive)
- Fluorescence diagnosis
- Ultrasonography (endometriomas)
- MRI (endometriomas, adhesions, masses)
- Immunoassays (follow-up to therapy)

TABLE 3.2

Common symptoms of endometriosis*

Symptom	Incidence (%)
Dysmenorrhea	60–80
Pelvic pain	30–50
Infertility	30–40
Dyspareunia	25–40
Menstrual irregularities	10–20
Cyclical dysuria/hematuria	1–2
Dyschezia (cyclic)	1–2
Rectal bleeding (cyclic)	< 1

* Reproduced with permission from Shaw RW. *An Atlas of Endometriosis*. Carnforth, Lancs: Parthenon, 1993

The depth of infiltration of endometriosis in the uterosacral ligaments and the rectovaginal septum is positively associated with pelvic pain and dyspareunia. Many of these patients also complain of pain during bowel motion while menstruating (dyschezia). Pain in the iliac fossae and flank may indicate involvement of the ureters, which may result in hematuria and dysuria. Rectal bleeding occurs in about 20% of patients who have significant bowel endometriosis. Very occasionally, if an endometrioma is ruptured or bleeds, acute abdominal pain is the presenting symptom. The disease may be found in abdominal scars from previous surgery (e.g. cesarean section) causing superficial cyclic pain, tenderness and swelling (Figure 3.1).

All types of abnormal bleeding from premenstrual spotting to oligomenorrhea and hypermenorrhea have been reported in patients; occasionally there may be atypical symptoms or normal bleeding. Rarely, endometriosis may present as massive and acute hemoperitoneum. Such cases can be caused by active bleeding of endometriosis of the fallopian tube, spontaneous rupture of vessels covering the uterine wall, pregnancy complicated by endometriosis and

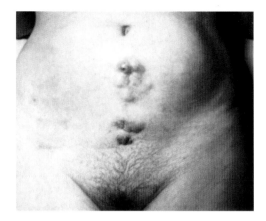

Figure 3.1 Endometriosis of an abdominal scar in a woman of 49 with a long history of the disease. Within 6 years it changed from benign to malignant. Reproduced with permission from Jeffcoate N. *Principles of Gynaecology*. 4th edn. London: Butterworth–Heinemann, 1975.

bleeding endometriotic implants and rupture of the uterine artery by erosion from an endometriotic lesion.

Physical examination

Pelvic endometriosis should be suspected if any of the following specific or non-specific findings are encountered during pelvic examination:

- multiple nodules along the uterosacral ligaments
- adnexal masses that may represent endometriomas
- rectovaginal endometriosis, which may be palpated by combined rectal and vaginal examination
- retroversion of the uterus, especially when it is fixed in position
- tenderness in the cul-de-sac in the absence of palpable pathology.

Differential diagnosis

It is important to be aware of the clinical diagnoses that can mimic endometriosis (Table 3.3). For example, endometriosis is commonly misdiagnosed as pelvic inflammatory disease (PID), and the true diagnosis is made only after repeated courses of antibiotics and laparoscopy. Endometriosis is also occasionally diagnosed as acute appendicitis.

TABLE 3.3

Differential diagnosis

Differential diagnosis of endometriosis and acute pelvic pain

- Pelvic inflammatory disease (PID)
- Acute appendicitis
- Ovarian cysts (rupture, torsion or infection)
- Ectopic pregnancy

Differential diagnosis of endometriosis and chronic pelvic pain

- Chronic pelvic inflammatory disease
- Adhesions as a result of previous surgery or infection
- Pelvic congestion syndrome
- Intermittent torsion of ovarian cyst
- Colitis and diverticulitis
- Chronic lumbosacral pain

The diagnosis should always be suspected if a patient complains of any of the typical symptoms of endometriosis, and it is important to recognize the possibility of the diagnosis if the symptoms are atypical.

Investigation and evaluation

Laparoscopy. This is the most important method for evaluation of the pelvis and should be considered the gold standard when endometriosis is suspected (Table 3.4). The accuracy of the diagnosis is dependent upon the skill of the laparoscopist and the thoroughness of the examination. Spots of endometriosis may be treated as soon as they are found (Figure 3.2). The following findings are possible.

Peritoneal and retroperitoneal endometrial implants may be typical or atypical. Typical pigmented lesions are dark powder-burn nodules surrounded by a fibrotic, thickened peritoneal patch. Endometriosis is confirmed on biopsy in 80–90% of cases. Non-pigmented atypical endometriosis can be the only manifestation in over half of patients. Jansen and Russell describe six types of atypical lesions: red, flame-like

TABLE 3.4

Laparoscopic examination

- Systematic and thorough evaluation of the pelvis
- Second puncture probes and other instruments to be used as routine
- Aspiration of all peritoneal fluid
- Lysis of adhesions
- Mobilization of the ovaries from the pelvic side wall
- Use of rectal and vaginal probes
- Recording of the location, appearance and extent of the disease
- Routine video recording of the procedure
- Thorough examination of all atypical lesions (e.g. white nodules, translucent blebs, red flame-like appearance)

lesions, translucent glandular lesions, subovarian adhesions, yellow-brown peritoneal patches, circular peritoneal defects and white opacified peritoneum, often thickened and raised.

Endometriosis-induced adhesions. The revised ASRM classification (Figure 1.7) provides a convenient framework for assessment, description and recording of adhesions. It is particularly important to evaluate lesions on the ovaries and fallopian tubes. Prognosis for infertility is related to the percentage of the surface covered with adhesions.

Endometriomas. Endometriomas are smooth-walled, dark brownish cysts. On incision, dense, brown, chocolate-like fluid is released. Occasionally, endometriomas may be confused with corpus hemorrhagicum or rarely with ovarian carcinoma. Ovarian punctures may aid in the detection of small and deep endometriomas.

Endometrioma of the bowel. This occurs most often on the rectum and sigmoid colon and in the cecum, appendix and terminal ileum. It is present in patients with severe endometriosis and is particularly important in patients with gastrointestinal symptoms.

Microlaparoscopy. This technique has the additional advantage of being minimally invasive. With the development of 2-mm laparoscopes

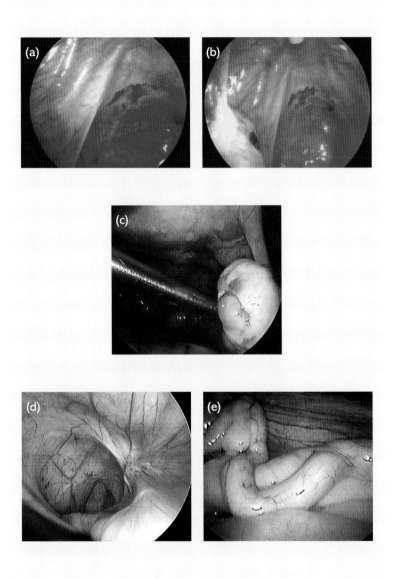

Figure 3.2 (a) Laparoscopic appearance of an untreated lesion.

(b) The same lesion after laser treatment. The brown marks are the laser burns.

(c) Right ovary showing superficial ovarian endometriosis.

(d) Pelvic sidewall superficial endometriosis.

(e) Endometriosis of the appendix and pelvic side wall.

with adequate visualization, diagnostic and operative procedures could be accomplished by microlaparoscopy in selected cases. In adolescents, microlaparoscopy can be very useful for evaluation of the pelvis, leaving no scars and no sutures.

Fluorescence diagnosis of endometriosis. The intraoperative diagnosis of endometriosis, especially minimal and mild endometriosis, is often extremely difficult. The ascertainment of non-pigmented changes in the peritoneal area is important, as these areas represent active forms of endometriosis. Marcoux and colleagues showed that patients with minimal or mild endometriosis benefit from surgical intervention. Therefore, an efficient therapeutic approach warrants a sufficient diagnosis in these patients, as simple laparoscopy is unreliable. Malik and colleagues introduced a new research tool for the diagnosis of endometriosis. Endometriotic lesions can be identified after application of 5-aminolevulinic acid and subsequent illumination with light of a certain wavelength, called fluorescence diagnosis. Refinement of this research might bear fruit in the future in terms of accurate diagnosis.

Imaging techniques. Selective use of imaging techniques, such as ultrasonography and MRI, can help to establish the extent of disease so that treatment can be planned. Other techniques (e.g. plain radiography and CT scanning) usually yield non-specific findings, but may be useful if endometriosis is suspected in the pleura or the bowel.

Ultrasonography should be performed using the transvaginal approach. The reliability of ultrasound depends on the nature of the lesions. In the detection of endometriomas, ultrasound is reported to have a sensitivity of 80% and specificity of 95%. In contrast, the sensitivity of ultrasound in detection of focal implants is poor and may be as low as 10%.

Typically, endometriomas are visualized as predominantly cystic masses with thick walls, often with diffuse acoustic enhancement or scattered internal echoes (Figure 3.3). Occasionally, endometriomas may contain septae, dependent echoes or fluid levels.

The diagnostic accuracy of ultrasound may be enhanced by Doppler flow studies. The blood flow in endometriosis is usually pericystic,

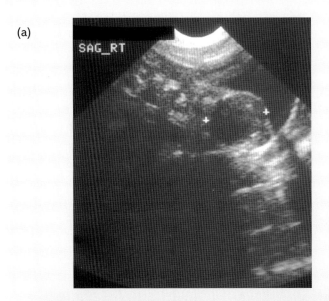

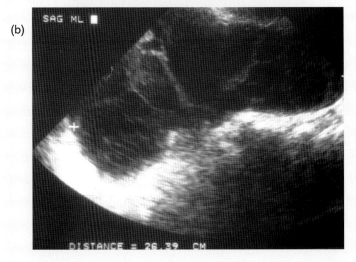

Figure 3.3 Ultrasound scans of ovarian endometrioma with 'ground-glass' appearance. (a) Scan of complex cystic right adnexal mass. (b) Scan of a large complex multiseptated mass. Images by kind permission of Dina Ragheb MD, Jane Clayton MD and Carlos Gimenez MD, Department of Radiology, Louisiana State University.

especially noticeable in the hilar region and usually visualized in regularly spaced vessels. Typically, the flow has a resistance index above 0.45. A scoring system that includes clinical parameters, CA-125 (see 'Immunoassays'), ultrasound and color Doppler flow results in outstanding reliability, with both sensitivity and specificity above 99%.

MRI detects endometriomas, ovarian adhesions and extraperitoneal masses (Figure 3.4). It may be useful in noting changes in size and number of endometriotic lesions during therapy, in detecting invasion of nerves (as in sciatic endometriosis) and in identifying abdominal wall lesions. MRI findings do not correlate with the stage of the disease.

Identification of endometriosis by MRI relies on the interpretation of pigmented hemorrhagic lesions. The signal characteristics vary according to the age of the hemorrhage. Typically, the lesion appears hyperintense on T1-weighted images and hypointense on T2-weighted images (owing to the presence of deoxyhemoglobin and methemoglobin). Identification of small implants may be better achieved with T1-weighted fat-suppressed images rather than with standard T1- and T2-weighted images. Gadolinium-enhanced imaging has not been useful in providing further diagnostic information.

Immunoassays. Three serum immunoassays have been tried in the diagnosis of endometriosis: CA-125, placental protein 14 (PP14) and antibodies to endometrium. Of these, CA-125 shows the most promise.

CA-125 is an ovarian epithelial tumor antigen that is detected by a monoclonal antibody designated OC-125. The incidence of elevated CA-125 levels increases with the severity of the disease, and mean concentrations correlate clearly with disease stage. However, because CA-125 levels are not elevated in mild forms of endometriosis, and do rise during and immediately after menstruation, CA-125 is not useful as a screening test, although it could be valuable in monitoring the effects of therapy. However, the development of a second-generation assay has prompted renewed interest, and the assay has been successfully used in conjunction with other examinations (e.g. ultrasonography).

Aromatase P450 messenger RNA expression. Aromatase P450, the enzyme that catalyzes the conversion of C19 steroids (androstenedione

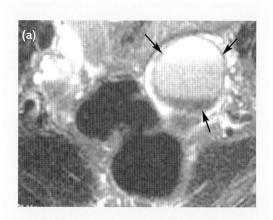

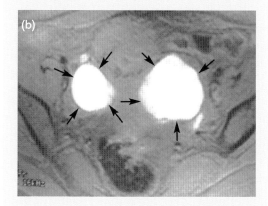

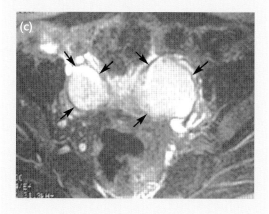

Figure 3.4 MRI images.
(a) Axial T2-weighted image of a rounded complex lesion in the left hemipelvis.
(b) Axial T1-weighted image of bilateral rounded lesions in the pelvis with increased signal consistent with endometriomas containing proteinaceous fluid.
(c) Axial T2-weighted image of bilateral rounded adnexal lesions with heterogeneous fluid signal intensity consistent with proteinaceous fluid within the endometriomas.
Images by kind permission of Dina Ragheb MD, Jane Clayton MD and Carlos Gimenez MD, Department of Radiology, Louisiana State University.

and testosterone) to estrone, is expressed in the eutopic endometrium of women with endometriosis but not in the endometrium of disease-free control subjects. It has been suggested that detection of aromatase P450 protein could be used as an outpatient screening test for endometriosis. However, endometrial aromatase P450 has also been associated with adenomyosis, leiomyomata and endometrial carcinoma. Furthermore, a recent prospective multicenter study has demonstrated that the relative high incidence of false negative results and lack of specificity would probably hinder clinical application.

Key points – Diagnosis of endometriosis

- Endometriosis is a syndrome of reproductive age, but may occur in adolescents owing to Müllerian malformations or in menopausal women receiving hormone replacement therapy.
- Dysmenorrhea, pelvic pain, infertility and dyspareunia are common symptoms of endometriosis.
- Pelvic pain and dyspareunia are strongly associated with the depth of implants of the uterosacral ligament and of the rectovaginal septum.
- The classic physical findings are fixed retroversion, nodules along the uterosacral ligaments and adnexal masses.
- Acute pain should be differentiated from acute appendicitis, pelvic inflammatory disease (PID), torsion or rupture of ovarian cyst and ectopic pregnancy.
- Chronic pain should be differentiated from chronic PID, adhesions, pelvic congestion syndrome, colitis and diverticulitis.
- Laparoscopy remains the gold standard for the diagnosis of pelvic endometriosis; fluorescence may enhance the accuracy still further.
- Ultrasound is invaluable in the diagnosis and follow-up of ovarian endometrioma.
- Magnetic resonance imaging detects endometriomas, adhesions and extraperitoneal masses.

New diagnostic tests have been developed based on simultaneous analysis of an endometrial biopsy and a peripheral blood sample. The MetrioTest, for example, was developed on the basis of a clinical study that compared T- and B-lymphocytes, natural killer cells, and macrophages in the endometrium of 173 patients with endometriosis and 195 normal controls. Future research is ongoing in this important area of diagnosis.

Key references

Brosens J, Timmerman D, Starzinski-Powitz A, Brosens I. Noninvasive diagnosis of endometriosis: the role of imaging and markers. *Endometriosis. Obstet Gynecol Clin N Am* 2003;30:95–114.

Dheenadayalu K, Mak I, Gordts S. Aromatase P450 messenger RNA expression in eutopic endometrium is not a specific marker for pelvic endometriosis. *Fertil Steril* 2002;78:825–35.

Duleba AJ. Diagnosis of endometriosis. *Endometriosis. Obstet Gynecol Clin N Am* 1997;24: 331–46.

Fauconnier A, Chapron C, Dubuisson JB et al. Relation between pain symptoms and the anatomic location of deep infiltrating endometriosis. *Fertil Steril* 2002;78: 719–26.

Gomel V, Taylor PJ. Diagnostic Laparoscopy in Infertility. In: Keye W, Chang RJ, Rebar RW et al., eds. *Infertility – evaluation and treatment.* Philadelphia: WB Saunders, 1995: chapter 24, 330–48.

Gleicher N, Karande V, Rabin D et al. The bubble test: A new tool to improve the diagnosis of endometriosis. *Hum Reprod* 1995;10:923.

Harada T, Kubota T, Aso T. Usefulness of CA19-9 versus CA125 for the diagnosis of endometriosis. *Fertil Steril* 2002;78:733–9.

Janicki TI, David L, Skaf R. Massive and acute hemoperitoneum due to rupture of the uterine artery by erosion from an endometriotic lesion. *Fertil Steril* 2002;78:879–81.

Jansen RP, Russell P. Nonpigmented endometriosis: Clinical, laparoscopic, and pathologic definition. *Am J Obstet Gynecol* 1986;155:1154–9.

Koninckx PR, Meuleman C, Demeyere S et al. Suggestive evidence that pelvic endometriosis is a progressive disease, whereas deeply infiltrating endometriosis is associated with pelvic pain. *Fertil Steril* 1991;55:759.

Malik E. Fluorescence diagnosis of endometriosis. In: Simon C, Smith SK, eds. *New Advances in the Pathogenesis and Management of Endometriosis.* Endometriosis Pre-congress course. Lausanne, Switzerland: European Society of Human Reproduction and Embryology, July 2001:57–61.

Rizk B. Microlaparoscopy in evaluation of the infertile patient. In: Almeida OD Jr., ed. Microlaparoscopy. New York: Wiley–Liss, 2000:chapter 10, 69–77.

Vignali M, Infantino M, Matrone R. Endometriosis: novel etiopathogenetic concepts and clinical perspectives. *Fertil Steril* 2002;78:665–78.

Medical treatment remains the cornerstone of the management of symptoms associated with endometriosis. In adolescents repeated courses of medical therapy will be needed to achieve symptom regression and avoid repeated surgery.

Hormonal therapy

This has been the main medical treatment for endometriosis for half a century. In the 1940s and 1950s, diethylstilbestrol and methyltestosterone were used, but were abandoned because the side effects were too great. In the 1960s, progestogen alone or combined estrogen/progestogen preparations were used in an attempt to produce a state of pseudopregnancy (see below), but again significant side effects rendered the treatment unpopular.

The modern era of hormonal therapy began with the description of danazol by Dmowski et al. in 1971. By 1987, the aggregate pregnancy rate was 40% in 16 studies involving 511 patients with mild endometriosis. However, Evers found the pregnancy rates to be similar to placebo-treated patients in randomized clinical trials, as verified by Collins. The concept of downregulation with GnRH agonist in endometriosis was introduced in 1984 from Quebec City in a pivotal paper by Lemay.

More recently, GnRH antagonists and antiprogesterones have been used, with favorable reports. Aromatase inhibitors are the newest class of medication with the greatest promise for the treatment of endometriosis. In the future, the development of antiangiogenesis therapy and matrix metalloproteinase inhibitors will have a marked impact on the treatment of endometriosis.

Pseudopregnancy. In 1959, Kistner reported the use of Enovid (norethynodrel and mestranol) in 58 women with pelvic endometriosis. It was a landmark in the history of pharmacological treatment of endometriosis, but it lost popularity because of both estrogenic and progestational side effects.

Danazol is a synthetic by-product of testosterone with a half-life of 4.5 hours. Peak levels are reached 2 hours after oral ingestion, and after 8 hours it is no longer detectable. It is metabolized in the liver, and the principal metabolite methylethisterone exhibits mild progestational and androgenic activity.

Danazol has a direct effect on steroidogenesis, including cholesterol cleavage enzymes, and on intracellular steroid receptors. It has an indirect action by decreasing GnRH pulse frequency, which may suppress ovulation.

Side effects. The most common are related to the hyperandrogenic state – weight gain, oily skin and hair, nausea, acne, muscle cramps, hot flashes and hirsutism. Deepening of the voice, though uncommon, is irreversible.

Danazol has multiple metabolic side effects, the most important of which relate to blood cholesterol. It decreases HDL and increases LDL levels, which must be taken into account as the drug is given for long periods (6–9 months). Its use should be avoided in women with a history of liver disease.

Gestrinone is a progesterone agonist/antagonist that has been used in Europe for treatment of endometriosis, but is unavailable in the USA. Gestrinone causes amenorrhea and endometrial atrophy, as do other androgen steroid analogs (e.g. danazol). It acts both centrally and peripherally to reduce estradiol and obliterate the mid-cycle luteinizing hormone (LH) surge.

Gestrinone has a long half-life, allowing oral administration 2–3 times weekly. In randomized clinical trials, gestrinone was effective in reducing the painful symptoms of endometriosis.

Side effects. Gestrinone has similar androgenic symptomatic and metabolic effects to danazol, but fewer hypoestrogenic side effects.

Progestogens. The effect of progestogens on endometrial tissue depends on the dosage, length of treatment and activity of the individual progestogen (Table 4.1).

Side effects include irregular vaginal bleeding, weight gain, fluid retention, breast tenderness and mood changes.

TABLE 4.1

Progestogens used in the treatment of endometriosis

Progestogens alone	Dose
Oral medroxyprogesterone acetate	2.5–20 mg daily
Injectable medroxyprogesterone acetate i.m.	50 mg/month or 150 mg every 3 months
Norethindrone (norethisterone)	2.5–20 mg/day
Megestrol acetate (rarely used in USA)	10–50 mg/day
Dydrogesterone (rarely used in USA)	10 mg 2–3 times daily

Progestogens in combination with estrogens	Dose
Desogestrel + ethinyl estradiol	0.15 mg/day and 0.02 mg/day respectively p.o. for 21 days of each 28-day cycle over 6 months
Cyproterone acetate	12.5 mg/day for 6 months

GnRH agonists. Native GnRH is a short-acting decapeptide that is secreted episodically into the pituitary circulation to regulate the release of LH and follicle-stimulating hormone (FSH). Continuous exposure to GnRH leads to downregulation of pituitary function, which suppresses ovarian steroid production, inducing a reversible pseudomenopause (Figure 4.1). Long-acting agonist analogs of GnRH capitalize on these effects. The medications must be given parenterally and are available as a nasal spray (nafarelin, buserelin), subcutaneous pellet (goserelin) or depot injection (leuprolide/leuprorelin; Table 4.2). All these medications help to reduce pain associated with endometriosis.

Clinical experience using GnRH agonist for symptomatic endometriosis has become extensive over the last 2 decades. Several investigators have expanded the utility of GnRH agonist in the treatment of endometriosis. Hornstein and colleagues specifically addressed 3 clinical areas. Firstly, they showed the efficacy of shorter (3-month) courses of GnRH agonist therapy. Secondly, they demonstrated the efficacy of retreatment of endometriosis using

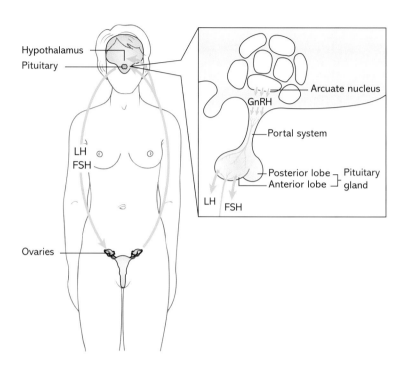

Figure 4.1 Gonadotropin-releasing hormone (GnRH) is secreted primarily into the portal circulation by the arcuate nucleus. It is then carried to the gonadotrope cell in the anterior pituitary, where it stimulates the synthesis, storage and release of luteinizing hormone (LH) and follicle-stimulating hormone (FSH).

GnRH agonist. Finally, they conducted a prospective randomized study to demonstrate that postoperative GnRH agonist enhances the effect of laparoscopic surgery on pain and significantly prolongs the time between surgery and the need for significant additional medical or surgical therapy to more than twice the period for placebo patients (Figure 4.2).

Side effects are most commonly hypoestrogenic, such as hot flashes. Bone loss may occur and bones may take 6–12 months to recover when treatment is completed.

GnRH agonist add-back therapy. In 1992, Barbieri proposed the estrogen threshold hypothesis, which highlighted the observation that decreased estradiol produced changes in bone mineral density (BMD), lipids, vasomotor symptoms, vaginal epithelium and endometrium. The

TABLE 4.2

Reduction in pain scores after treatment with GnRH analog leuprolide (leuprorelin)

	Depot leuprolide injection		Placebo		Significance
	n	Mean change in pain score	n	Mean change in pain score	
Dysmenorrhea	28	−2.2	21	−0.2	$p < 0.001$
Pelvic pain	28	−1.2	21	−0.3	$p = 0.001$
Dyspareunia	17	−0.4	13	0.1	ns
Pelvic tenderness	28	−1.0	21	-0.3	$p = 0.001$

Data from Dlugi AM et al. 1990

magnitude of alteration varies between tissue systems as shown in Figure 4.3. No significant loss in BMD occurs until the estradiol level

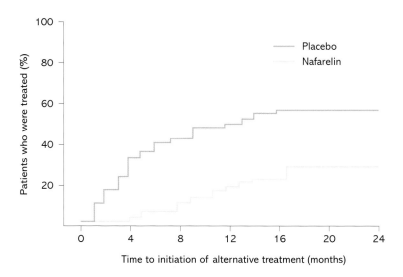

Figure 4.2 Time to initiation of alternative treatment for patients who were treated postsurgically with nafarelin versus placebo. Data from Lemay et al. 1999.

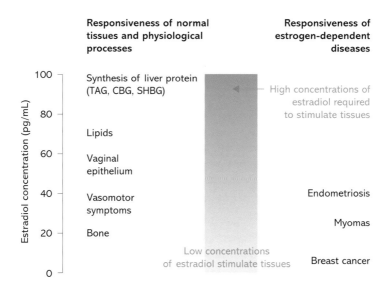

Figure 4.3 Variation in sensitivity to estradiol of normal and disease processes. Data from Barbieri 1992.

has sunk to 20 pg/mL. Vasomotor symptoms begin at about 40 pg/mL or less and vaginal epithelium starts to become atrophic at 60 pg/mL or less. Treatment regimens for certain diseases have different threshold estradiol levels. Symptomatic endometriosis requires the serum level of estradiol to be below 40 pg/mL. This therapeutic window will vary from woman to woman, but in general, the range of circulating estradiol should be between 30 and 50 pg/mL. A therapeutic window of estradiol level which will minimize the risk of a decrease in BMD but will not compromise the treatment of endometriosis is the ideal goal. Therefore, to counter the adverse impact of prolonged hypoestrogenism, GnRH agonists can be used with add-back therapy in various regimens (Figure 4.4). Those of proven efficacy for treatment of endometriosis include progestogen alone, progestogen and estrogen combinations, or progestogen and bisphosphonates.

Both the 17-hydroxyprogesterone derivative (Provera) and 19-nortestosterone derivative (norethindrone in the USA and norethisterone in the UK) have an established ability to promote endometrial atrophy (pseudopregnancy). In this sense, the addition of progestogen only to a long-term GnRH regimen provides a multi-modality attack on the pathophysiology of endometriosis.

In terms of the impact on bone density, progestogen-only add-back therapy was found to be sufficient to eliminate the GnRH-induced decrease in radial bone density (as shown by single-photon absorptiometry). Similarly, combinations of nafarelin and norethindrone/norethisterone or histrelin and medroxyprogesterone acetate proved fully protective for the lumbar spine (as shown by dual-photon absorptiometry). In contrast, treatment with histrelin and norethindrone/norethisterone failed to protect from GnRH-induced decrease in lumbar bone density. The use of depot leuprolide (also called leuprorelin) in conjunction with norethindrone/norethisterone,

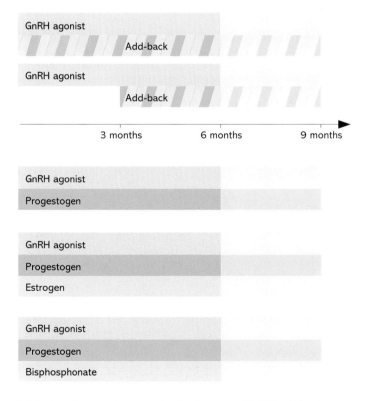

Figure 4.4 Options for gonadotropin-releasing hormone (GnRH) add-back regimen to protect bones while the disease is treated.

5–10 mg daily, was associated with a decrease in lumbar bone density of 2.7% after 6 months' therapy. Both norethindrone/norethisterone and medroxyprogesterone acetate combat the symptom of hot flashes.

GnRH antagonists have been studied by Kupker et al. to determine the feasibility of using a subcutaneous injection of GnRH antagonist in the treatment of endometriosis. Diagnostic laparoscopy before GnRH antagonist administration showed a mean Stage III endometriosis. All patients (15/15) reported no symptoms (including hot flashes, mood swings, loss of libido or vaginal dryness) during the treatment. Serum estradiol oscillated around a mean of 50 pg/mL. Regression occurred in 60% (9/15) of cases, and the degree of endometriosis declined to Stage II (Figure 4.5). This study demonstrated that sequential administration of GnRH antagonist, cetrorelix administration once

(a)

(b)

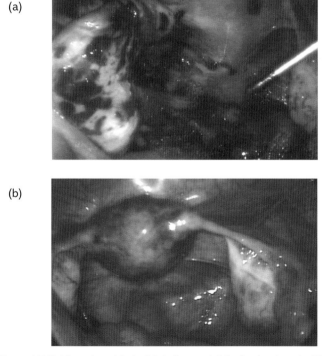

Figure 4.5 Pelvic endometriosis (a) before and (b) after treatment with cetrorelix. Reproduced with permission from Kupker et al. 2002.

weekly over 8 weeks, creates a new opportunity for medical treatment for symptomatic endometriosis preserving basic estrogen production. The authors' theory is that preserving basic estrogen production during the course of treatment does not influence the regression of endometriosis but still helps in alleviating the major side effects of suppression seen when GnRH agonist is given alone without add-back therapy.

Selective estrogen receptor modulators (SERMs). Raloxifene is a nonsteroidal SERM developed primarily to treat postmenopausal osteoporosis. It is the most widely tested SERM to date: more than 10 000 women have been enrolled in clinical trials of the prevention and treatment of osteoporosis. Raloxifene acts as an estrogen agonist in some tissue and an estrogen antagonist in other types, such as reproductive tissue.

Two studies have examined raloxifene treatment of endometriosis in animal models, and the data are encouraging. Raloxifene has been studied in healthy women of reproductive age; the sonographic and progesterone values were typically ovulatory. Therefore, in women of reproductive age, raloxifene does not prevent ovulation, tends to increase estrogen concentration and produces a minimal antiestrogenic effect on the endometrium. On this basis, raloxifene would not seem to be effective in treating endometriosis, an estrogen-responsive disorder in which endometrial proliferation at least of ectopic tissue must be strongly suppressed.

Antiprogesterones. Mifepristone, known as RU-486, has been used for pregnancy termination and other medical indications. It has been shown both to inhibit ovulation and to disrupt endometrial integrity, and has been used in trials in patients with symptomatic endometriosis to induce chronic anovulation.

In two pilot studies, RU-486, 100 mg/day, was given for 3 months with significant improvement in pelvic pain, though there was no visible regression of endometriosis; in a follow-up study, treatment was extended to 6 months and the dose lowered to 50 mg/day, with a significant decrease in pelvic pain within 4 weeks.

These pilot studies indicate a potential role for antiprogesterones in the treatment of endometriosis. More than 400 different antiprogesterone analogs have been synthesized over the last decade.

Selective progesterone receptor modulators could potentially selectively suppress estrogen-dependent endometrial growth and induce reversible amenorrhea without the adverse systemic side effects of estrogen deprivation. Several selective progesterone receptor modulators are now available. J867 has been shown to suppress both menses and endometrial proliferation effectively, while CDB (VA) induces inhibition of endometrial proliferation alone. It has been suggested that selective progesterone receptor modulators might be used in the treatment of both endometriosis and uterine leiomyomata.

Aromatase inhibitors. The development and growth of endometriosis is estrogen-dependent. In contrast to the eutopic endometrium, the endometriotic tissues have several molecular aberrations that favor increased local levels of 17β-estradiol. A positive feedback mechanism has been identified that is responsible for continuous formation for both 17β-estradiol and prostaglandin E2 through upregulation of aromatase and cyclooxygenase-2 (Cox-2) in endometriotic stromal cells. Furthermore, levels of 17β-estradiol are further increased in endometriotic tissue by impaired inactivation because of deficient 17β-hydroxysteroid dehydrogenase type II expression in endometriotic epithelial cells. These findings are the molecular basis for treating endometriosis with aromatase inhibitors (Figure 4.6). The potent and selective third-generation non-steroidal aromatase inhibitors anastrozole and letrozole have substantial advantages over earlier agents in terms of efficacy and tolerability.

Side effects. The side effects of aromatase inhibitors include mild headache, nausea, and diarrhea. Hot flashes occur infrequently. Letrozole and anastrozole are associated with less weight gain and dyspnea, fewer thromboembolic events and less vaginal bleeding than megestrol acetate and other progestins. The long-term effects of these drugs on bone mineral density and serum lipids are unknown.

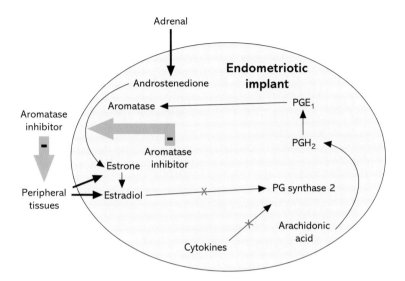

Figure 4.6 The molecular basis for treatment for endometriosis with an aromatase inhibitor. Modified from Bulun et al. 1999.

The first report of treatment of severe endometriosis with an aromatase inhibitor has been published by Bulun and colleagues. A 57-year-old woman who presented with recurrent severe endometriosis after hysterectomy and bilateral salpingo-oophorectomy was evaluated. Two additional laparatomies were performed because of severe pelvic pain and bilateral ureteral obstruction giving rise to left renal atrophy and right hydronephrosis. Recurrent pelvic endometriosis was evident from a 30-mm vaginal lesion that did not respond to an oral megestrol acetate treatment over 4 months. Anastrozole, 1 mg/day, was given orally. Alendronate and calcium were also given daily. The lesion decreased from 30 to 3 mm by the end of 9 months' treatment. Pain rapidly decreased and completely disappeared after the second month of treatment. The markedly high pretreatment levels of aromatase P-450 mRNA in the endometriotic tissue had become undetectable in a rebiopsy specimen after 6 months of treatment. The circulating levels of serum β–estradiol were reduced by 50% and the bone density by 6%. This was the first successful report on the treatment of severe endometriosis in postmenopausal women. Hence, postmenopausal women with endometriosis, in whom the estimated prevalence of the disease has been reported to be about 2%, may benefit from therapy with the new aromatase inhibitors. The full potential of these drugs in the treatment of endometriosis is currently under investigation.

Immunomodulators and anti-inflammatory agents

Vignali et al. recently reviewed the role of immunomodulators and anti-inflammatory agents in the treatment of endometriosis (Table 4.3). Four compounds with immune-enhancing properties have been investigated in the treatment of endometriosis: cytokines interleukin-12 and interferon-α-2b, and two synthetic immunomodulators, the guanosine analog loxoribine and the acetylcholine nicotinic receptor

TABLE 4.3

Immunomodulators and anti-inflammatory agents tested for the treatment of endometriosis

Drug	Type
Agents that enhance cell-mediated immunity	
Interleukin-12	Cytokine
Interferon-α-2b	Cytokine
Loxoribine	Synthetic immunomodulator
Levamisole	Synthetic immunomodulator
Agents that reduce inflammation	
Diclofenac	NSAID
Ibuprofen	NSAID
Mefenamic acid	NSAID
Celecoxib, rofecoxib, valdecoxib	NSAIDs (Cox-2 inhibitors)
Danazol	Synthetic androgen
Pentoxifylline	Methylxanthine derivative
Recombinant human TNF binding protein-1	

NSAID, non-steroidal anti-inflammatory drug; TNF, tumor necrosis factor
Modified from Vignali et al. 2002

agonist levamisole. These compounds are known to be pleiotropic stimulators of the components of the immune system.

Because the clinical profile of endometriosis is typical of inflammatory disease, therapy with anti-inflammatory or cytokine drugs has been proposed. Non-steroidal anti-inflammatory drugs are useful in the treatment of painful menstruation associated with endometriosis. Ibuprofen and naproxen have been found to improve symptoms significantly. Celecoxib and valdecoxib inhibit prostaglandin synthesis by the selective inhibition of Cox-2 and are efficacious in the relief of dysmenorrhea in patients with endometriosis.

Antiangiogenesis therapy

VEGF is currently considered to act as a major mediator in the pathogenesis of endometriosis by promoting angiogenesis. VEGF is produced in large quantities by hypoxic endometrial cells during the menstrual phase and by activated macrophages in the menstrual effluent and peritoneal cavity. Menstrual blood can induce similar responses in the peritoneum, thus facilitating adhesion of endometrial cells and neoangiogenesis. Antiangiogenesis therapy has been tested in rodents; the future challenge is to adapt it for humans.

Suppression of matrix metalloproteinases inhibits the establishment of ectopic lesions by human endometrium in nude mice, and also in adenomyosis.

The next challenge is treating endometriosis by nonhormonal methods to selectively prevent the development of endometriosis or to suppress existing endometriosis without suppressing ovulation.

Key points – Medical treatment of endometriosis

- Medical treatment is a key component of the management of chronic pain associated with endometriosis; most patients have used most if not all types of medication.
- Gonadotropin-releasing hormone (GnRH) agonists have been the most efficacious medical treatment over the past 15 years; oral contraceptives and NSAIDs are the most widely used therapies.
- Repeated short courses of GnRH agonists are helpful in the management of pain linked to endometriosis.
- Postoperative GnRH therapy may prolong the time to the next intervention.
- Add-back therapy with GnRH agonists helps patients to tolerate the menopausal side effects and prevents bone loss.
- GnRH agonist downregulation before in-vitro fertilization (IVF) may improve IVF outcome in patients with severe disease and good ovarian reserve.
- Progestogens are efficacious for the treatment of endometriosis.
- GnRH antagonists have been used successfully in the treatment of endometriosis, but are not first-line therapy.
- Aromatase inhibitors have been successful in postmenopausal women and are now being tested in premenopausal women.
- Non-steroidal anti-inflammatory drugs and Cox-2 inhibitors alleviate the dysmenorrhea and pain associated with endometriosis.
- Antiangiogenesis therapy and matrix metalloproteinase inhibitors are likely to be the therapies of the future.

Key references

Agarwal A. Differential effects of
GnRH agonist therapies: implications
regarding the estrogen threshold
hypothesis. In: Lemay A, Maheux R,
eds. *Understanding and Managing
Endometriosis: Advances in Research
and Practice*. New York: Parthenon,
1999:chapter 30, 199–204.

Barbieri RL. Hormonal therapy
of endometriosis: the oestrogen
threshold hypothesis. *Am J Obstet
Gynecol* 1992;166:740–5.

Bergquist A. Effects of triptorelin
versus placebo on the symptoms
of endometriosis. *Fertil Steril*
1998;69:702–8.

Brosens I. Pathophysiology and
medical treatment of endometriosis
associated infertility. In: Seibel MM,
ed. *Infertility: A Comprehensive
Text*. Stamford: Appleton & Lange,
1997:189–202.

Bulun SE, Zeitoun K, Takayama L.
Aromatase expression in
endometriosis: biology and clinical
perspectives. In: Lemay A, Maheux
R, eds. *Understanding and Managing
Endometriosis: Advances in Research
and Practice*. New York: Parthenon,
1999:chapter 20, 139–48.

Corson SL. *Endometriosis: The
Enigmatic Disease*. Durant, Canada:
Essential Medical Information
Systems, 1992.

Dlugi AM, Miller JD, Knittle J.
Lupron depot (leuprolide acetate for
depot suspension) in the treatment of
endometriosis: a randomized,
placebo-controlled, double-blind
study. Lupron Study Group. *Fertil
Steril* 1990;54:419–27.

Edmonds DK. Add-back therapy in
the treatment of endometriosis: the
European experience. *Br J Obstet
Gynecol* 1996;103:10–13.

Evers JLH. The pregnancy rate of the
no-treatment group in randomized
clinical trials of endometriosis
therapy. *Fertil Steril* 1989;52:906–7.

Henzl MR, Corson SL, Moghissi K
et al. Administration of nasal
nafarelin as compared multicenter
double-blind comparative clinical
trial. *N Engl J Med* 1988;318:485–9.

Hornstein MD. Expanding the utility
of the GnRH agonists in the
treatment of endometriosis. In:
Lemay A, Maheux R, eds.
*Understanding and Managing
Endometriosis: Advances in Research
and Practice*. New York: Parthenon,
1999:chapter 31, 205–9.

Kettel LM, Murphy AA, Morales AJ
et al. Treatment of endometriosis
with the antiprogesterone
mifepristone (RU486). *Fertil Steril*
1996;65:23.

Kettel LM, Murphy AA, Mortola JF et al: Endocrine responses to long-term administration of the antiprogesterone RU486 in patients with pelvic endometriosis. *Fertil Steril* 1991;56:402.

Kupker W, Felberbaum RE, Krapp M et al. Use of GnRH antagonists in the treatment of endometriosis. *Reprod BioMed Online* 2002;5:12–16.

Lemay A, Maheux R, Faure N et al. Reversible hypogonadism induced by a luteinizing hormone-releasing hormone (LHRH) agonist (Buserelin) as a new therapeutic approach for endometriosis. *Fertil Steril* 1984;41: 863–871.

Moghissi KS. Add-back therapy in the treatment of endometriosis: the North American experience. *Br J Obstet Gynecol* 1996;103:14.

Vignali M, Infantino M, Matrone R et al. Endometriosis: novel etiopathogenetic concepts and clinical perspectives. *Fertil Steril* 2002;78:665–78.

5 Surgical treatment of endometriosis

Surgery is used for the diagnosis and treatment of endometriosis. The choice of procedure depends on the stage of endometriosis, the site of the disease and whether the patient desires to have a child. The objectives of surgery are to:

- relieve symptoms
- restore fertility
- remove endometriotic implants
- delay recurrence of the disease.

Conservative surgery: laparoscopic surgery

The major advantage of laparoscopy is that it allows diagnostic and therapeutic procedures (Table 5.1) to be performed at the same time, with minimal and gentle manipulation of tissues to avoid trauma. If endometriosis is found it should be ablated or removed, preferably by means of laser surgery to reduce tissue damage. It is also possible to combine assisted conception techniques with treatment of the disease.

TABLE 5.1

Laparoscopic procedures for treatment of endometriosis

- Adhesiolysis
- Removal of ovarian endometriomas
- Oophorectomy
- Resection of bladder endometriosis
- Resection of ureteric endometriosis
- Resection of invasive bowel endometriosis
- Appendectomy
- Laparoscopic-assisted vaginal hysterectomy
- Laparoscopic uterosacral nerve ablation
- Laparoscopic presacral neurectomy

The principles of laparoscopic surgery for endometriosis are:
- eradication of all visible disease by removal, vaporization or destruction
- biopsy of ovarian cystic lesions or suspect areas before laser application
- thorough examination of the peritoneal cavity and ovarian lesions before the cyst is entered
- restoration of normal anatomy
- complete hemostasis.
  Laparoscopy is indicated in women with:
- infertility of more than a year's duration
- pelvic pain unresponsive to medical treatment for 3–6 months
- adnexal masses that may indicate endometriomas.

Laparoscopic treatment of ovarian endometriomas. Several treatments have been described for the laparoscopic management of ovarian endometriomas (see Chapter 6). The cyst wall is opened laparoscopically and the 'chocolate' material aspirated. As the wall is almost invariably adherent to the ovarian tissue, destruction of the wall is achieved by laser vaporization starting from the bottom and moving towards the top in a spiral fashion (Figure 5.1). Where the cyst is not adherent to the ovary, it is stripped intact by hydrodissection or by sharp dissection (Figure 5.2). Superficial and residual endometriotic spots should be treated by CO_2 laser ablation.

Conservative surgery: adjunctive procedures for pelvic pain
The surgical technique used to treat pelvic pain will depend on where the pain occurs.

Uterine suspension. This is usually performed to prevent recurrence of adhesions in the cul-de-sac and to minimize dyspareunia from central endometriosis. It corrects fixed retroversion of the uterus and allows better access of the fallopian tubes to the pouch of Douglas (Figure 5.3).

Laparoscopic uterosacral nerve ablation (LUNA). This procedure is likely to benefit patients with significant central dysmenorrhea. It will not

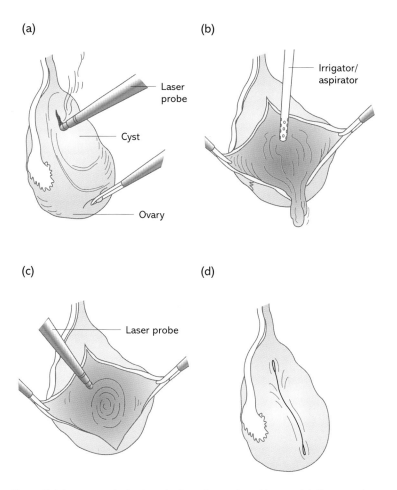

(a)

Laser probe

Cyst

Ovary

(b)

Irrigator/
aspirator

(c)

Laser probe

(d)

Figure 5.1 Laparoscopic treatment of ovarian endometriomas: (a) the ovary is grasped and the cyst opened with a laser; (b) the cyst is washed out with physiological saline so the cyst wall can be examined; (c) the laser probe destroys the cyst wall, starting from the bottom and moving outwards in a spiral fashion; (d) the cyst edges fold towards each other with no need for suturing.

benefit those with lateral pelvic pain or pain of gastrointestinal or urinary tract origin. It also has no benefit in terms of treating infertility. It should not be performed if the anatomy of the ureters and cul-de-sac is unclear.

In 1989, Ruggi performed the first interruption of uterosacral ligaments. In 1955, Doyle, in a landmark article, studied the results of

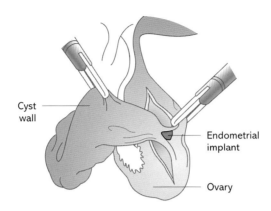

Cyst
wall

Endometrial
implant

Ovary

Figure 5.2 Laparoscopic view of the cyst wall being separated from the ovarian cortex.

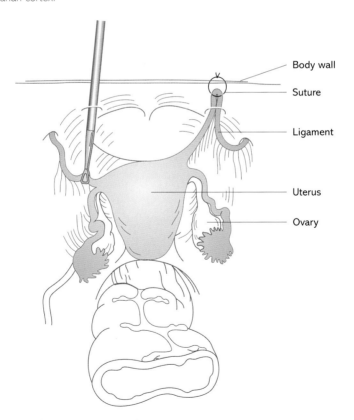

Body wall

Suture

Ligament

Uterus

Ovary

Figure 5.3 Laparoscopic view of uterine suspension.

vaginal or abdominal transection of the uterosacral ligaments for the treatment of dysmenorrhea and found that over 70% of patients had pain relief. In a controlled double-blind study using electrocoagulation, Lichten and Bombard reported significant relief of menstrual pain in 9 of 11 patients who had a LUNA procedure, compared with none who underwent diagnostic laparoscopy only. In 1989, Sutton demonstrated an 86% improvement rate in 100 women with endometriosis and 73% in 26 women with primary dysmenorrhea after laparoscopic surgery and LUNA.

Study of laparoscopic treatment of endometriosis and pelvic pain. It is well established that there is no correlation between the ASRM classification of endometriosis and pelvic pain. Sutton and colleagues performed the first randomized, double-blind, placebo-controlled trial in patients with Stage I, II or III endometriosis (r-ASRM classification; see Figure 1.7) at laparoscopy. Patients with Stage IV disease were excluded by the institute's Institutional Review Board because they felt it was unethical to withhold treatment from patients at this stage. The patients were randomized to have either a diagnostic laparoscopy with the removal of peritoneal fluid or laser ablation of all visible lesions and uterosacral nerve ablation. The patients and the nurses were blinded as to which procedure had been undertaken.

It is very interesting that at 3 months there was no difference in pain between the two groups. At 6 months, 63% of those patients who had LUNA experienced relief of their symptoms, while only 23% of those patients who had the diagnostic procedure alone were better. Only 38% of patients with Stage I disease improved after operative intervention, whereas 69% and 100% of patients with Stage II and Stage III disease respectively were better. When these patients were followed up 1 year later, 56% of patients still had some relief and 44% were still suffering despite aggressive surgical intervention. The conclusion is that more than 40% of patients will still have pain after aggressive surgery, and surgery should be considered as cytoreductive and palliative rather than curative.

Presacral neurectomy. This procedure (Figure 5.4) is used to treat patients with midline pelvic pain. It can be performed by laparotomy

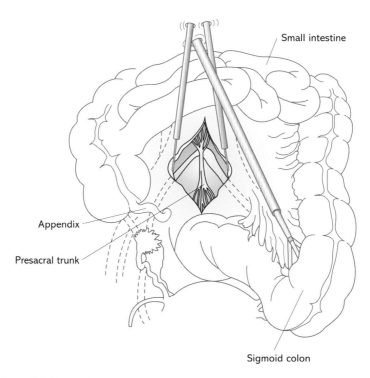

Figure 5.4 Presacral neurectomy.

or by laparoscopy, though the latter is demanding. There is no evidence that the procedure enhances fertility or affects menstruation.

Laparoscopic presacral neurectomy is accomplished using high-resolution laparoscopy and a video camera. Five puncture sites are usual, with a fan retractor to move the rectosigmoid colon. The presacral nerve bundles are identified, dissected free and elevated.

A variety of techniques are used for excision, including endoloop suture ligation with excision of the intervening nerve bundles, bipolar cauterization of the nerve bundles with resection of the intervening segment, or a combination of bipolar cautery and Nd-YAG laser.

The main complications are bleeding from the middle sacral or inferior mesenteric vessels and injury to the ureter, though other problems have been reported including bladder dysfunction, constipation and vaginal dryness, as well as painless labor. The overall success of the procedure exceeds 50%.

Second-look laparoscopy is an appropriate procedure in patients who have undergone laparoscopy for the resection of endometriosis or who may have residual pain. It is usually scheduled several weeks after the initial surgery to check whether any endometriotic spots were missed, and allows separation of the de novo adhesions that are still relatively filmy in consistency. It also provides an opportunity to assess the prognosis for fertility.

Laparoscopic treatment of bladder and bowel endometriosis. These techniques are employed at specialist centers. Nezhat and colleagues recently reported on the laparoscopic management of 15 patients with infiltrating endometriosis of the bladder with great success.

Radical surgery

In the early days, surgical removal of the uterus was the sole treatment for endometriosis. Nowadays it is seldom indicated and is usually reserved for patients with intractable pain who have completed their family or for women in whom conservative surgery has failed. At least 12% of all endometriosis patients require radical surgery.

Definitive surgery offers prompt and long-term relief of pain compared with medical treatment. Most hysterectomies are performed by the abdominal route although, in selected cases, if laparoscopy reveals a free cul-de-sac or allows lysis of adhesions, then laparoscopic-assisted vaginal hysterectomy can be performed safely and effectively.

The number of hysterectomies performed for endometriosis increased steadily from the 1960s to 1990s, far more so than for other diagnoses. In the USA, endometriosis was the primary indication for hysterectomy in 20% of white women and 9% of black women.

Total abdominal hysterectomy with or without bilateral salpingo-oophorectomy. The decision to remove or conserve the ovaries should be individualized. In young women with less extensive disease and no involvement of the bladder or bowel, the ovaries may be conserved. older women with extensive pelvic disease, the ovaries are usually removed. In the USA, total abdominal hysterectomy alone was the typical surgery in the older series, and bilateral salpingo-oophorectomy has become more common in the more recent series. The age of the patient also has an impact: bilateral salpingo-oophorectomy was performed at the time of hysterectomy in 52% of women 44 years of age or younger, and in 81% of women 45 years of age or older.

Pelvic pain was documented following hysterectomy with and without ovarian conservation by Namnoum and colleagues. Uterosacral ligaments were not routinely resected at the time of hysterectomy. Compared with women who underwent oophorectomy, women who had a hysterectomy with preservation of ovaries had a 6.1-fold greater risk of developing pain and an 8.1-fold greater risk of reoperation. The recurrence of symptoms and reoperations after total abdominal hysterectomy with and without bilateral salpingo-oophorectomy is discussed in Chapter 9.

Laparoscopically assisted vaginal hysterectomy. During vaginal hysterectomy, endometriotic nodules may be out of view or technically impossible to remove. Even during abdominal hysterectomy, subtle implants of endometriosis are often missed. As a result, the patient's pain may persist despite hysterectomy and salpingo-oophorectomy. Since implants can be identified easily by laparoscopy owing to the magnification of the pelvic surfaces, they can be destroyed by laser or excised before the removal of the uterus or ovaries. Complete laparoscopic removal of pelvic endometriosis before vaginal hysterectomy is more likely to alleviate the patient's symptoms than simple hysterectomy alone.

Surgical management of endometriosis in the uterosacral ligaments. Horowitz and colleagues suggested that recurrent pain following hysterectomy may be due to persistent endometriosis in the uterosacral ligaments. These authors routinely resected the uterosacral ligaments even in their conservative management of endometriosis. Many patients who did not have gross disease on the peritoneal surface did, in fact, have deep retroperitoneal invasion of the uterosacral ligament, occasionally extending toward the sacrum. 75% of their patients reported decreased or no discomfort after completion of this procedure. The remaining 25% had the same or increased pain, probably secondary to irritable bowel syndrome.

Transrectal ultrasonography has been used to image the invasion of the rectovaginal septum; involvement was present in one-third of the extensive cases. These patients would benefit from radical resection of the uterosacral ligaments, usually performed by laparotomy, as shown by Horowitz and colleagues, or laparoscopically, as advocated by Chapron and colleagues from France and Reich in the USA.

Key points – Surgical treatment of endometriosis

- Surgery should relieve symptoms, restore fertility, remove endometrial implants and delay recurrence.
- Radical surgery, including hysterectomy, is now reserved for women who have completed their families.
- If possible, at least one ovary should be preserved in young women.
- Laparoscopic surgery is indicated in women with infertility of one year's duration, pelvic pain that does not respond to medical therapy, or adnexal masses.
- Ovarian endometriosis can be treated laparoscopically by ovarian cystectomy or cyst drainage and ablation of the cyst wall by laser or thermocoagulation.
- Recurrence of pain following hysterectomy may be due to residual disease in the uterosacral ligaments.
- Laparoscopic uterosacral nerve ablation helps to alleviate pain in patients with dysmenorrhea and central pelvic pain.
- Intractable central pelvic pain is treated with laparoscopic presacral neurectomy.

Key references

Canis M, Bruhat MA, Pouly JL. Techniques for ablation and excision of endometriosis. In: Nezhat CR, Berger GS, Nezhat FR et al., eds. *Endometriosis: Advanced Management and Surgical Techniques*. New York: Springer, 1995:chapter 10, 85–94.

Chapron C, Camus M. *Reproductive Surgery*. Endometriosis Pre-congress course. Lausanne, Switzerland: European Society of Human Reproduction and Embryology, July 2001.

Hesla JS, Rock JA. Endometriosis. In: Rock JA, Thompson JD, eds. *TeLinde's operative gynecology*, 8th edn. Philadelphia: Lippincott–Raven, 1997:chapter 27, 585–624.

Hornstein MD, Hemmings R, Yuzpe AA et al. Use of nafarelin versus placebo after reductive laparoscopic surgery for endometriosis. *Fertil Steril* 1997;68:860–4.

Kim AH, Adamson GD. Results of surgical therapy for endometriosis. In: Gershenson DM, Olive DL, eds. *Operative techniques in gynecologic surgery: Surgery for endometriosis*, vol 2. Philadelphia: WB Saunders, 1997:122–9.

Markham SM, Rock JA. Adjunctive procedures in treatment of endometriosis: LUNA presacral neurectomy, and uterine suspension. In: Nezhat CR, Berger GS, Nezhat FR et al., eds. *Endometriosis: Advanced Management and Surgical Techniques*. New York: Springer, 1995:chapter 13, 117–26.

Namnoum AB, Gehlbach DL, Hickman TN et al. Incidence of symptom recurrence after hysterectomy for endometriosis. *Fertil Steril* 1995;64:898–902.

Nezhat C, Nezhat F, Nezhat C et al. Laparoscopically assisted vaginal hysterectomy, laparoscopic hysterectomy, and bilateral salpingo-oophorectomy. In: Nezhat CR, Berger GS, Nezhat FR et al., eds. *Endometriosis: Advanced Management and Surgical Techniques*. New York: Springer, 1995:chapter 17, 173–188.

Reich H, McGlynn F, Salvat J. Laparoscopic treatment of cul-de-sac obliteration secondary to retrocervical deep fibrotic endometriosis. *J Reprod Med* 1991;36:516–22.

Sutton CJG, Ewen S, Whitelaw N et al. Prospective, randomized, double-blind controlled trial of laser laparoscopy in the treatment of pelvic pain associated with minimal, mild or moderate endometriosis. *Fertil Steril* 1994;62:696–700.

The management of infertility associated with endometriosis is outlined in Figure 6.1. There are several approaches to treatment:
- surgical
- medical
- expectant (i.e. no treatment)
- combined medical and surgical.

In a meta-analysis by Adamson and Pasta of all the studies in the English-language literature since 1977, interventions consisted of no

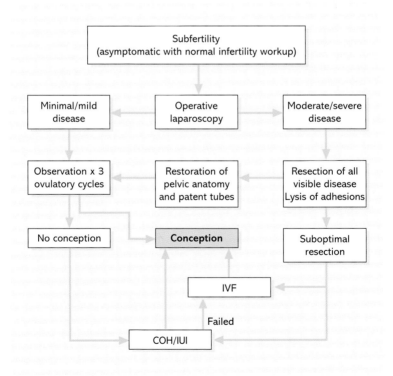

Figure 6.1 Algorithm for the management of patients with infertility caused by endometriosis.

treatment, medical treatment or surgical treatment by laparoscopy or laparotomy; the results are depicted in Figure 6.2.

Surgical treatment

Surgical versus non-surgical approaches. Endoscopic treatment of endometriosis-associated infertility is the standard practice. The surgical approach (laparoscopy or laparotomy) is significantly superior to non-surgical treatment (no treatment or medical treatment) for all stages of infertility associated with endometriosis. A meta-analysis of data comparing surgical with non-surgical treatment showed the surgical approach increased pregnancy rates by 38%, and confidence intervals were 28–48% higher (Figure 6.3). Collins, in an elegant review, confirmed the place of surgery at the present time in the management of endometriosis-associated infertility from early reports as well as the cohort studies and a single randomized clinical trial.

Early reports were promising because the treatments did not delay conception. As early as 1979, Hasson reported better fertility in 19 patients with electrocoagulation. The next year, 40 of 100 consecutive

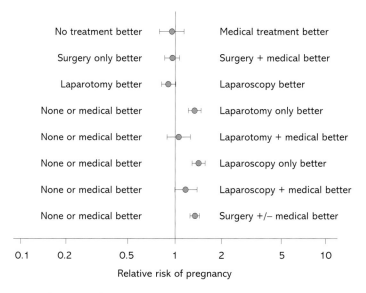

Figure 6.2 Summary of combined Mantel–Haenszel meta-analysis estimates of endometriosis treatment. Data from Adamson and Pasta 1994.

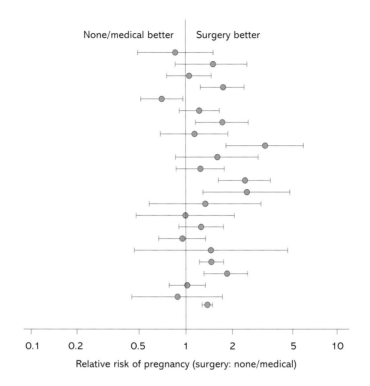

Figure 6.3 Meta-analysis of data comparing surgical with non-surgical treatment of endometriosis-associated infertility. The surgical approach is favored, with crude pregnancy rates 38% higher than for non-surgical treatment. Data from Adamson and Pasta 1994.

patients treated with laparoscopy conceived. The results of coagulation and vaporization were similar in a study completed in 1987.

Cohort studies. Comparative studies, including five cohort and one alternate assignment, showed a 2.7-fold higher pregnancy rate after surgery. However, the studies showed methodological weaknesses, suggesting that clinical practice should not be altered until the results of randomized clinical trials are available.

The Canadian endometriosis prospective randomized clinical trial.
There are few well-designed trials of the effectiveness of surgical procedures, but the planners of the ENDOCAN study designed a

superb model for enrolment efficiency and follow-up. The study recruited infertile women contemplating laparoscopy and, if endometriosis was diagnosed, the long-distance telephone random allocation system was activated so that destruction of the lesion could be initiated within a minute or diagnostic laparoscopy could be completed without treatment of the endometriosis. Follow-up was maintained for 36 weeks; the primary outcome was pregnancy at 20 weeks. Women without endometriosis were followed and all women were encouraged to avoid co-interventions. The study showed a relative benefit of ablation of lesions of 1.7 (95% CI 1.2–2.6). The cumulative 20-week pregnancy rate at 36 weeks was 30.7% in laparoscopic surgery patients and 17.7% in diagnostic laparoscopy patients (Figure 6.4). The monthly fecundity rate was 4.7 and 2.4 per 100 person-months, respectively.

This important study has several implications, as listed by the Canadian authors.

- The absolute increase in pregnancy attributable to laparoscopic surgery is 13%. Stated differently, one in eight women with minimal or mild endometriosis should benefit.
- Operative laparoscopy adds little time, carries fewer risks and can be done on an outpatient basis. Therefore, ablation or resection should be performed at the time of diagnostic laparoscopy.
- The monthly fecundity rate after laparoscopic surgery is much lower than expected in fertile women. This means that the destruction of implants and adhesiolysis does not cure all the factors by which endometriosis contributes to infertility, or that factors other than endometriosis interfere with infertility.

Laparoscopy or laparotomy? The laparoscopic approach has been popularized because of significant improvement in equipment and operative techniques. Adamson and colleagues carried out a life-table analysis of patients with minimal or mild endometriosis, but with no other infertility factors. They found similar outcomes for laparoscopy and laparotomy. For moderate or severe disease, laparoscopy had better pregnancy results than laparotomy. Therefore, dependent on the individual situation, the primary surgical approach should be

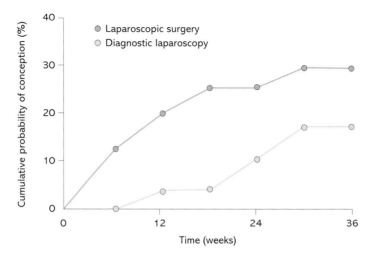

Figure 6.4 Cumulative probability of a pregnancy carried beyond 20 weeks in the 36 weeks after laparoscopy in women with endometriosis. Data from Marcoux et al. 1997.

laparoscopy, which offers the following advantages over laparotomy:

- better visualization
- less tissue trauma
- less adhesion formation
- shorter recovery time
- equivalent, if not better, success rates.

Ovarian endometriomas. As previously stated, there are several techniques for the surgical management of ovarian endometriomas. They can be removed by laparoscopic excision or laparoscopic drainage followed by electrocoagulation or laser treatment. Simple drainage has no place in the management of fertility. Laparoscopic treatment of ovarian endometriomas resulted in pregnancy rates of 50% (26 of 52) and 52% (12 of 23) in two studies by Reich and McGlynn and by Wood et al.

Randomized clinical trial of laparoscopic ovarian cystectomy versus drainage and ablation. A recent randomized clinical trial by Beretta and colleagues compared ovarian cystectomy with drainage and coagulation. The pregnancy rate was increased following ovarian cystectomy relative to drainage and coagulation (67% versus 23.5%). Although the numbers are small, the study is the first prospective randomized study comparing cystectomy to drainage. Some authors propose ovarian cystectomy in every case because histological analysis of endometriotic lesions shows 4% atypical lesions in some cases. These lesions could be a risk factor for developing cancer. On the other hand, an important argument against cystectomy is the absence of a real cleavage plane between the endometriotic cyst and the ovarian cortex.

Laparoscopic management of endometriomas prior to IVF. When carefully selected and appropriately applied, laparoscopic ovarian cystectomy or laparoscopic drainage and vaporization will not impair the response during IVF. This will be discussed in detail in Chapter 7.

Ovarian endometriomas: laparoscopy or laparotomy? Adamson et al. addressed this question in a prospective cohort study comparing the treatment of endometrioma by laparoscopy or laparotomy. They found comparable estimated cumulative pregnancy rates at 3 years (52% for laparoscopy and 46% for laparotomy, Figure 6.5). With improved techniques, laparoscopy has become the standard approach for drainage and excision of endometriomas, with these observations:

- recurrence rate is approximately 10%
- de novo adhesion formation is approximately 20%
- incidence of recurring adhesions is approximately 80%
- normal ovarian function is retained after conservative surgery.

Endometriosis in the posterior cul-de-sac and rectovaginal septum. In a study by Reich and colleagues, laparoscopic surgery for partial or complete cul-de-sac obliteration resulted in a 74% pregnancy rate. However, over one-third of the patients required more than one laparoscopy. In another study by Adamson and colleagues, life-table pregnancy rates for patients with complete posterior cul-de-sac obliteration was 29.6% for those treated laparoscopically, compared with 23.7% for those treated by laparotomy.

Medical treatment

Medical therapy alone does not improve fertility potential. The data from randomized controlled studies have been homogeneous despite

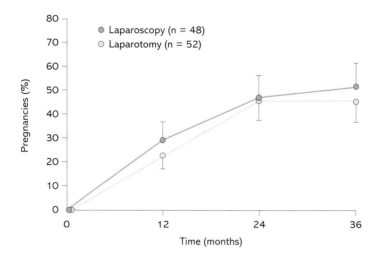

Figure 6.5 Estimated cumulative life-table pregnancy rates for laparoscopy vs laparotomy for the treatment of endometriomas. Reproduced with permission from Adamson GD, Subak LL, Pasta DJ et al. Comparison of CO_2 laser laparoscopy with laparotomy for treatment of endometriomata. *Fertil Steril* 1992;57:965–73.

different interventions and designs. The additional costs and side effects render the medical option inadvisable in patients with endometriosis-associated infertility.

There is one important exception to the lack of efficacy of medical treatment: long-term downregulation using GnRH agonist before in-vitro fertilization. To date, there are three studies that confirm such efficacy, and these will be discussed in Chapter 7.

However, medical therapy is very effective in reducing the pain associated with endometriosis. Generally, 80–90% of patients receiving GnRH agonists or other treatment will experience significant improvement in the disease, and recurrence rates correlate with the severity of the disease. The side effects of treatment are the most important factor in choosing a particular medical therapy.

Expectant management

The biggest disadvantage of medical treatment for minimal endometriosis associated with infertility is that it induces anovulation for 6–9 months, therefore preventing these women becoming pregnant. Expectant management (i.e. doing nothing) is adopted by many to good effect (Table 6.1).

Combined medical and surgical treatment

Malinak has observed a cycle in the popularity of medical versus surgical treatment of endometriosis over the years. It is currently common practice for the therapies to be used concurrently to treat the disease.

Theoretically, preoperative medical treatment should have the following advantages:

- it facilitates surgical technique
- it reduces pelvic vascularization and inflammation
- it increases the pregnancy success rate
- it lowers the risk of recurrence of the disease
- it prevents delay between surgery and attempt at pregnancy.

TABLE 6.1

Expectant management in patients with infertility and mild endometriosis

Study	n patients	n pregnancies	Pregnancy (%)	Pregnancy rate (%/month)
Garcia and David (1977)	17	11	64.7	5
Schenken and Malinak (1982)	18	13	72.2	10.2
Siebel et al. (1982)	28	14	50.0	1.11
Portuondo et al. (1983)	31	19	61.2	8.3
Olive et al. (1985)	34	13	52.9	5.7
Hull et al. (1987)	56	21	37.5	
Bayer et al. (1988)	36	17	47.2	
Total	220	108	49.1%	

Theoretically, postoperative medical therapy should have the following advantages:

- it cures residual disease following surgery
- it does not mask the effect of preoperative treatment.

Meta-analysis of combined medical and surgical therapy. A meta-analysis by Adamson et al. of data from studies between 1984 and 1993 found that medical therapy after surgery is no better than laparoscopy or laparotomy alone (relative risks 0.97; 95% CI 0.87–1.09); Vercellini et al. likewise demonstrated equivalent pregnancy outcome (Figure 6.6). The homogeneity of the studies in this comparison strengthens the conclusion that no difference exists. Also, the costs, the side effects and delayed fertility argue against any role for medical therapy in the postoperative period. Data are insufficient to perform a meta-analysis on preoperative medical treatment.

In conclusion, medical treatment does not add to the benefits of surgical treatment of endometriosis for infertility. Three controlled trials

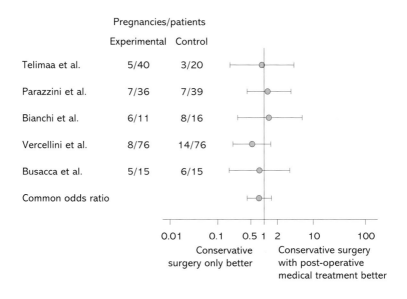

Figure 6.6 Combined data from controlled studies demonstrating that conservative surgery with postoperative medical therapy is not better than conservative surgery alone in infertility outcome. Data from Vercellini et al. 2003.

have been published comparing postoperative medical therapy to surgery alone. None of these trials have proved that fertility outcome could be improved. However, the addition of postoperative GnRH agonist has been shown in at least one randomized study to delay the clinical recurrence of pain from endometriosis.

Key points – Treatment of infertility associated with endometriosis

- Infertility linked to endometriosis has been treated surgically, medically, with both techniques combined, and expectantly.
- The surgical approach, whether by laparotomy or laparoscopy, is superior to medical or expectant management at all stages of the disease.
- Endoscopic treatment of endometriosis-associated infertility is the standard.
- In minimal or mild endometriosis, a higher pregnancy rate is achieved after ablation.
- Laparoscopic surgery has equivalent or better success rates compared with laparotomy, as well as having several practical advantages.
- Pregnancy rates are lower for medical therapy alone than for surgery, and postoperative medical therapy does not improve the outcome after surgery.
- Gonadotropin-releasing hormone agonist downregulation before in-vitro fertilization may improve the pregnancy outcome in patients with advanced endometriosis and good ovarian reserve.

Key references

Adamson GD, Pasta DJ. Surgical treatment of endometriosis-associated infertility: Meta-analysis compared with survival analysis. *Am J Obstet Gynecol* 1994;171: 1488–505.

Hughes E, Fedorkow DM, Collins JA. A quantitative overview of controlled trials in endometriosis-associated infertility. *Fertil Steril* 1993;59:963–70.

Marconi G, Vilela M, Quintana R et al. Laparoscopic ovarian cystectomy of endometriomas does not affect the ovarian response to gonadotropin stimulation. *Fertil Steril* 2002;78:876–81.

Marcoux S, Maheux R, Berube S. Laparoscopic surgery in infertile women with minimal or mild endometriosis. Canadian Collaborative Group on Endometriosis. *N Engl J Med* 1997;337:217–22.

Metzger D. Treatment of infertility associated with endometriosis. In: Nezhat CR, Berger GS, Nezhat FR et al., eds. *Endometriosis: Advanced Management and Surgical Techniques*. New York: Springer, 1995:chapter 25, 245–55.

Reich H, McGlynn F, Salvat J. Laparoscopic treatment of cul-de-sac obliteration secondary to retrocervical deep fibrotic endometriosis. *J Reprod Med* 1991;36:516–22.

Schenken RS. Treatment of human infertility: the special case of endometriosis. In: Adashi EY, Rock JA, Rosenwaks Z, eds. *Reproductive endocrinology, surgery and technology*, vol 2. Philadelphia: Lippincott–Raven, 1996.

Vercellini P, Frontino G, De Giorgi O et al. Endometriosis: preoperative and postoperative medical treatment. *Obstet Gynecol Clin N Am* 2003; 30:163–80.

Assisted reproductive technology and endometriosis

While medical treatment of endometriosis is successful in terms of relief of pain and symptoms, no controlled studies have shown its efficacy in improving the outcome of infertility. However, for those patients with endometriosis who have undergone medical or surgical therapy, or both, assisted reproductive technology (ART) offers hope. The techniques used include:
- controlled ovarian hyperstimulation (COH)
- intrauterine insemination (IUI)
- in-vitro fertilization (IVF)
- gamete intrafallopian transfer (GIFT)
- intracytoplasmic sperm injection (ICSI).

COH and IUI

Several studies have demonstrated the efficacy of COH and IUI. The advantages are substantial and include:
- increased number of oocytes available for fertilization
- higher levels of follicular and luteal phase gonadal steroids
- increased number of sperm present at the fertilization site
- optimized likelihood of gamete interaction between the oocytes and sperm.

The generally accepted rate of fecundity of normal couples is about 20%. In patients with endometriosis or unexplained infertility, the rate varies from 1% to 3%, depending on the age of the female partner, whether a pregnancy has previously been achieved and the duration of infertility. Haney and colleagues have shown that COH and IUI in women with endometriosis gives a cycle fecundity rate approaching the norm (Table 7.1), except in cases of severe endometriosis.

Results of studies.
- hMG (human menopausal gonadotropins) and IUI versus hMG and intercourse: MFR (monthly fecundity rate) in the IUI group was

TABLE 7.1

Controlled ovarian hyperstimulation and intrauterine insemination in women with endometriosis

Stage of endometriosis	n pregnancies/ n cycles	Cycle fecundity (%)
Minimal	45/280	16
Mild	14/143	10
Moderate	9/51	18
Severe	0/14	0
Total	68/488	14

Data from Haney et al. 1997

13%; for intercourse it was 7%.

- COH and IUI cycles versus expectant management: MFR for the COH and IUI group was 15%, while that in the expectant group 5%; cumulative pregnancy rates were 37% and 24%.
- Superovulation-intrauterine insemination (SO-IUI): The clinical pregnancy rate in patients was 20.5%; 96% of the pregnancies occurred in the first two cycles.
- Postsurgery patients in an hMG IUI treatment group demonstrated a constant fecundity rate until after 40 years of age. At 12 months after surgery, 57% aged under 35 years and 33% over 35 had conceived. By 24 months, 77% of patients under 35 had conceived, while 39% of those over 35 conceived. When hMG IUI was initiated 6 months after surgery in women over 35, 81% achieved pregnancy within 16 months of surgery. In contrast, when hMG IUI was started 12 months after surgery in women under 35 years, 88% achieved pregnancy compared with 77% not treated with hMG IUI.

We may conclude that hMG IUI improves infertility associated with endometriosis, taking into account surgery, age and stage of disease. Women aged 35 years or over, and women with moderate and severe disease, appear to benefit most from hMG IUI soon after surgery. Superovulation is an effective treatment for patients with endometriosis who have patent fallopian tubes.

IVF

In-vitro fertilization is an effective treatment of infertility associated with endometriosis. The timing of IVF depends on the age of the woman, duration of infertility and the presence or absence of other causes of infertility. The evidence presented in this sections shows that, in women with endometriosis who failed to conceive after surgery, IVF should offer a higher pregnancy rate than repeat surgeries. The use of GnRH agonist in a long protocol of ovarian stimulation leads to the highest pregnancy rate. The presence of endometriomas significantly increases the risk of infection.

Results of IVF in women with endometriosis compared with other causes of infertility. Although initial studies suggested that fertilization was reduced in women with endometriosis compared with tubal or unexplained infertility, subsequent, larger studies showed comparable fertilization rates. Recent results published by the Human Fertilization and Embryology Authority (HEFA) in the UK, the French National Registry and the US Society of Reproductive Technology (SART; combined results in Figure 7.1) showed no significant difference between IVF and embryo transfer in achieving pregnancy in patients with endometriosis and other indications associated with infertility. Pregnancy and birth rates achieved with IVF in women with different causes of infertility are shown in Table 7.2.

On the other hand, Barnhart and colleagues demonstrated in their recent meta-analysis on the effect of endometriosis on IVF that all aspects of IVF are negatively affected by the presence of endometriosis (Figure 7.2). A very important point is also made; namely, the SART analysis was not adjusted for confounding factors as was the meta-analysis. Controlling for confounding factors strengthened the negative associations in the meta-analysis, with the exception of the implantation rate, which remained unchanged.

IVF versus expectant management. Kodama analyzed the cumulative pregnancy rates in 60 patients who started their IVF cycle after operative laparoscopy and 58 patients who were managed expectantly without IVF treatment in Japan. The cumulative conception rates at

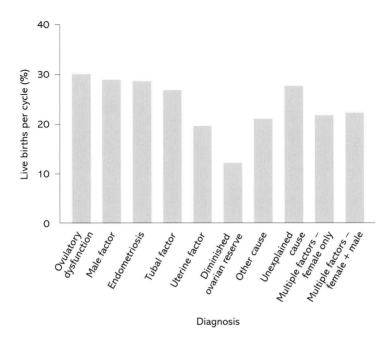

Figure 7.1 Live birth rates for women with endometriosis compared with other diagnoses after ART cycles with fresh non-donor eggs or embryos. Data from SART 1999.

TABLE 7.2

IVF clinical pregnancy and live birth rates for female causes of infertility

	n cycles	% of all cycles*	Clinical pregnancy rate	Live birth rate
Tubal disease	14 667	39.6	16.9	13.3
Endometriosis	3663	9.9	18.6	15.0
Unexplained	15 627	42.2	19.0	15.9

Data from UK Human Fertilization and Embryology Authority, 6th Annual Report
* Number of treatment cycles between 1 January 1995 and 3 March 1996.

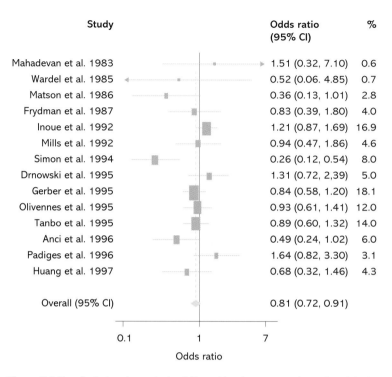

Study	Odds ratio (95% CI)	%
Mahadevan et al. 1983	1.51 (0.32, 7.10)	0.6
Wardel et al. 1985	0.52 (0.06. 4.85)	0.7
Matson et al. 1986	0.36 (0.13, 1.01)	2.8
Frydman et al. 1987	0.83 (0.39, 1.80)	4.0
Inoue et al. 1992	1.21 (0.87, 1.69)	16.9
Mills et al. 1992	0.94 (0.47, 1.86)	4.6
Simon et al. 1994	0.26 (0.12, 0.54)	8.0
Drnowski et al. 1995	1.31 (0.72, 2,39)	5.0
Gerber et al. 1995	0.84 (0.58, 1.20)	18.1
Olivennes et al. 1995	0.93 (0.61, 1.41)	12.0
Tanbo et al. 1995	0.89 (0.60, 1.32)	14.0
Anci et al. 1996	0.49 (0.24, 1.02)	6.0
Padiges et al. 1996	1.64 (0.82, 3.30)	3.1
Huang et al. 1997	0.68 (0.32, 1.46)	4.3
Overall (95% CI)	0.81 (0.72, 0.91)	

Odds ratio: 0.1 — 1 — 7

Figure 7.2 Unadjusted meta-analysis of the odds of pregnancy in endometriosis patients vs tubal factor patients as controls. Data from Barnhart et al. 2002.

36 months after laparoscopy were 62% in the IVF group and 43% in the control group; the difference is not statistically significant. For patients who conceived, the interval from laparoscopy to conception was statistically shorter in the IVF group than in the control group (20.6 ± 15.1 versus 27.1 ± 18.4 months, $p < 0.005$). For patients ≥ 32 years of age, the conception rates were higher in the IVF group (59% vs 27%, respectively). A relatively large, but not significant, difference in the conception rate between the IVF and controls was also observed in patients with Stage III or IV endometriosis (52% vs 27%). There was no impact of duration of infertility or gravidity on the cumulative conception rates.

IVF versus repeat surgery. A Canadian study compared IVF with laparoscopic reoperation in cases of moderate or severe endometriosis (Stage III and IV); the cumulative pregnancy rates 3, 7 and 9 months after laparoscopy were 5.9%, 18.1% and 24.4% respectively, compared with 33.3% and 69.6% after one and two cycles of IVF treatment, respectively. There was no difference in fertilization, implantation, pregnancy or live birth rates between patients with endometriosis and those with tubal infertility.

Implantation in IVF for endometriosis. Implantation rates in patients with endometriosis have been controversial. One retrospective study reporting the results of 35 patients who underwent 89 IVF cycles suggested that implantation was significantly lower in women with endometriosis compared with those with unexplained or tubal infertility. In a larger study of 140 patients who underwent 182 cycles, there was no difference in pregnancy rate per embryo transfer in women with endometriosis compared with couples with male-factor, unexplained or tubal infertility. There was also no difference in miscarriage rate.

Oocyte donation and endometriosis. When the results of oocyte donation in women with active endometriosis were compared with its use in women without endometriosis, there was no difference in pregnancy rate or implantation rates. These studies suggest that any putative adverse effect of endometriosis on the reproductive outcome is probably related to impaired oocyte or embryo quality. These findings also support the appropriateness of IVF for infertility associated with endometriosis. We fully agree with Buckett and colleagues that IVF is the best treatment for infertility associated with endometriosis.

IVF outcome in relation to stage of endometriosis. Although some early studies suggested that pregnancy rates were significantly lower in women with severe endometriosis than in those with mild or minimal endometriosis, more recent studies have shown no difference between rates in women with Stage III or IV disease and those with Stage I or II disease.

IVF outcome and ovarian stimulation protocols. While earlier studies suggested poor pregnancy rates after IVF in women with endometriosis, more recent studies suggest that the disease has no impact on the outcome. The introduction of GnRH agonist for downregulation before controlled ovarian hyperstimulation is a major reason for the change in the trend. It has been suggested that prolonged pituitary suppression with GnRH agonist before IVF improves pregnancy rates in women with severe endometriosis. More studies are required to confirm this.

Endometriomas and IVF. Endometriomas pose two problems in relation to the outcome of IVF. The first is the genuine concern that mechanical removal of the pseudocapsule of an endometrioma may impair ovarian reserve and its response to gonadotropin stimulation in IVF. The second issue is the risk of infection during IVF treatment.

Ovarian response after laparoscopic ovarian surgery prior to IVF. Determining the ideal surgical technique for the treatment of endometriomas remains controversial. Some investigators suggested the drainage of the content and lavage of the cavity followed by vaporization of the internal wall of the endometrioma by CO_2 laser. Recently, Donnez and colleagues reported that patients with endometriomas who underwent this surgical treatment had an ovarian response similar to that of patients with tubal factor infertility. Furthermore, in cases of single endometriomas, the surgically treated ovary had a similar response to the non-involved contralateral ovary. In a retrospective study, Marconi and colleagues evaluated the ovarian response during IVF/ET in patients who previously underwent laparoscopic removal of the pseudocapsule of the ovarian endometriomas. The control group consisted of patients of similar age undergoing IVF/ET for tubal factor infertility. There were no differences in the parameters studied including estradiol levels, oocytes retrieved, number and quality of embryos transferred and clinical pregnancy rate. The only difference was a significantly higher number of gonadotropin ampules needed for ovarian hyperstimulation.

In conclusion, these two studies confirmed that when appropriately applied, the two techniques of laparoscopic management of ovarian endometriomas do not affect the ovarian response during IVF/ET. The most important message is the comment by Marconi and colleagues about careful, gentle and selective bipolar coagulation of the bleeders. In a very recent study, Aboulghar and colleagues showed that the outcome of IVF is seriously impaired in patients who undergo aggressive surgical management of endometriosis, and made a plea for conservative surgical management.

The presence of endometriomas significantly increases the risk of infection following use of transvaginal oocytes for IVF. Several case reports have highlighted significant risk of pelvic abscess even with the prophylactic use of broad-spectrum antibiotics. Endometriomas should be removed laparoscopically before IVF; alternatively, they should be avoided during oocyte retrieval if possible.

IVF outcome in relation to age. The pregnancy rate achieved with IVF in women with endometriosis decreases with age as shown by the ten-year series from the Lister Hospital, London (Figure 7.3).

Cumulative conception rates in endometriosis. Tan et al. analyzed the cumulative conception and live birth rates in endometriosis in 5000

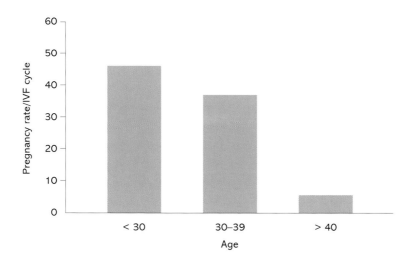

Figure 7.3 Pregnancy rate per IVF cycle related to age in patients with endometriosis. Data from Lister Hospital, UK.

consecutive cycles performed at the Bourn–Hallam Medical Center. There were no differences in the cumulative conception and live birth rates in patients with endometriosis and those with unexplained infertility. In the era of IVF prior to ICSI, Rizk and colleagues demonstrated that cumulative conception rates in 3505 IVF cycles were similar in couples with endometriosis to those in couples with tubal damage or unexplained infertility. They argued that the number of embryos replaced would depend on the age and quality of embryos rather than the cause of infertility.

Meta-analysis of IVF in endometriosis. Barnhart and colleagues performed a meta-analysis including 22 published studies on IVF in patients with endometriosis. A total of 2377 IVF cycles of women with endometriosis and of 4383 IVF cycles of women without endometriosis were included. The chance of achieving pregnancy was significantly lower in patients with endometriosis (odds ratio = 0.56, 95% CI 0.44–0.70) when compared with tubal factor controls (Figure 7.2). Multivariant analysis also demonstrated a decrease in fertilization, implantation rates and a significant decrease in the number of oocytes retrieved in endometriosis patients. Pregnancy rates in women with severe endometriosis were significantly lower than for women with mild disease (odds ratio = 0.60, 95% CI 0.42–0.87). In effect, the pregnancy rate in endometriosis is almost half that of women with other indications for IVF. The data suggest that the effect of endometriosis is not exclusively on the receptivity of the endometrium but also on the development of the oocyte and embryo.

GIFT

GIFT has been associated with a high pregnancy rate in patients with endometriosis. When GIFT is combined with laser treatment for the disease, success rates are even greater; for example, 45%/65% live birth/pregnancy rates as against 36%/34% in women not receiving concurrent treatment. The pregnancy rate was increased to 55% in women with minimal and mild endometriosis when a short course of GnRH was given before hMG stimulation.

ICSI

ICSI has become the most widely applied method of assisted fertilization for male infertility. A retrospective study assessed the impact of endometriosis on the outcome of ICSI: there was a significant reduction in the number of oocytes retrieved from women with endometriosis compared with those without, but there were no significant differences in either fertilization or pregnancy and implantation rates.

Key points – Assisted reproductive technology and endometriosis

- Assisted reproductive technology (ART) is an effective means of achieving pregnancy for infertile patients with endometriosis.
- ART includes controlled ovarian hyperstimulation, intrauterine insemination, in-vitro fertilization, intracytoplasmic sperm injection and gamete intrafallopian transfer.
- The monthly fecundity rate is 1–3% in patients with endometriosis, depending on their age and the duration of infertility.
- Controlled ovarian hyperstimulation and intrauterine insemination improve pregnancy rates compared with expectant management.
- In-vitro fertilization is the treatment of choice in patients who fail to conceive after laparoscopic surgery.
- In-vitro fertilization is more effective than repeat surgery or expectant management.
- Work with donated oocytes suggests that the quality of oocytes is a greater problem than implantation for in-vitro fertilization.
- Ovarian endometriomas larger than 3 cm should be treated laparoscopically before in-vitro fertilization; great care must be taken not to diminish the ovarian reserve.
- Gamete intrafallopian transfer is associated with high pregnancy rates in endometriosis patients with patent tubes. However, its role in general has greatly decreased.

Key references

Barnhart K, Dunsmoor-Su R, Coutifaris C. Effect of endometriosis on in vitro fertilization. *Fertil Steril* 2002;77:1148–55.

Buckett WM, Too LL, Tan SL. Treatment of endometriosis associated with infertility – IVF is the best treatment. In: Lemay A, Maheux R, eds. *Understanding and Managing Endometriosis: Advances in Research and Practice*. New York: Parthenon, 1999:chapter 24, 165–77.

Geber S, Ferreira DP, Prates LF et al. Effects of previous ovarian surgery for endometriosis on the outcome of assisted reproduction treatment. *Reprod BioMed Online* 2002;5:162–6.

Haney AF. Endometriosis. In: Lobo RA, Mishell DR, Paulson RJ et al., eds. *Mishell's Textbook of Infertility, Contraception and Reproductive Endocrinology*, 4th edn. Oxford: Blackwell Scientific, 1997:653–5.

Marcus SF, Edwards RG. High rates of pregnancy after long-term down-regulation of women with severe endometriosis. *Am J Obstet Gynecol* 1994:171;812–7.

Rizk B, Tan SL, Edwards RG. Cumulative pregnancy rates in IVF. British Fertility Society Annual Meeting, The London Hospital, London, December 1989.

Rizk B. Endometriosis and in vitro fertilization. *A Clinical Step-by-Step Course for Assisted Reproductive Technologies*. American Society for Reproductive Medicine. 35th Annual Postgraduate Program, 57th Annual Meeting, 2002:15–23.

Rizk B, Aksel S, Helvacioglu A. Gamete intrafallopian transfer in patients with pelvic endometriosis. *Gynecol Obstet Reprod Med* 1995;1:124–6.

Simon C, Gutierrez A, Vidal A et al. Outcome of patients with endometriosis in assisted reproduction: results from in-vitro fertilization and oocyte donation. *Hum Reprod* 1994;9:725–9.

Society of Assisted Reproductive Technology and Centers for Disease Control. Assisted reproductive technology success rates – national summary and fertility clinic reports, vol 2: Central US, 1995. Atlanta: RESOLVE, 1997.

Tan SL, Mason BA, Rizk B et al. The relation between age and etiology and success in in-vitro fertilisation. 7th World Congress on Human Reproduction, Helsinki, Finland, 1989.

Extrapelvic endometriosis is estimated to occur in 1–10% of patients with pelvic endometriosis. The disease has been reported in almost all body structures, but the most common sites are the intestine, urinary tract, distal areas in the abdominal cavity, lungs, skin and nervous system.

Gastrointestinal endometriosis

It is estimated that 7–37% of patients with endometriosis have bowel involvement. Up to 50% of those with severe endometriosis have gastrointestinal endometriosis, the most common sites being the rectosigmoid colon (50%), appendix (15%), small bowel (14%), rectum (14%) and the cecum and colon (5%) (Figure 8.1).

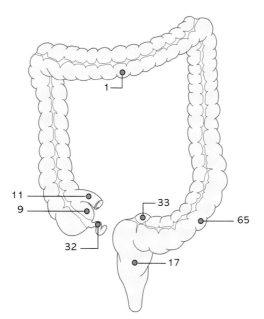

Figure 8.1 Sites of 168 lesions in 163 patients with endometriosis of the bowel. Data from Weed JC, Ray JE. Endometriosis of the bowel. *Obstet Gynecol* 1987;69:727–30.

The symptoms of gastrointestinal endometriosis are listed in Table 8.1.

Appendiceal involvement may present as an incidental finding with or without pelvic disease. The appendix should be inspected in all patients undergoing surgery for endometriosis, as should Meckel's diverticulum, and if it is found they should be removed.

Urinary tract endometriosis

Urinary tract endometriosis is thought to affect 1–4% of patients with pelvic endometriosis; there have also been many cases without pre- or postoperative evidence of pelvic disease.

The bladder is the most common site of endometriosis in the urinary tract (80–90% of cases), usually occurring in the trigone, dorsal wall, at the uterovesical junction or transmurally. Deeply infiltrating endometriosis rarely involves the bladder. From the histopathological point of view, the pathogenesis of bladder endometriosis is much debated. An intraperitoneal origin is the hypothesis most frequently proposed. Recently two other hypotheses were suggested. First, bladder endometriosis could be considered as a bladder adenomyosis as the consequence of metaplasia of müllerian remnants. Second, it could result from the extension of adenomyosis

TABLE 8.1

Symptoms of gastrointestinal endometriosis

- Diarrhea
- Constipation
- Perimenstrual changes in bowel habits
- Rectal bleeding
- Pain with defecation
- Tenesmus
- Abdominal distension
- Small-caliber stools
- Colicky abdominal pain

TABLE 8.2

Symptoms of urinary tract endometriosis

- Dysuria
- Frequency of urination
- Suprapubic pressure
- Back pain

lesions of the anterior uterine wall to the bladder. Chapron et al. recently completed a study on deep bladder endometriosis and found the anatomic pathological lesions to be heterogeneous; no hypothesis could be proposed as a single explanation for their pathogenesis.

The ureters are involved in 10–15% of cases, with the left being more commonly affected than the right; ureteral lesions are usually found in the distal third of the ureter below the pelvic brim. Ureteral obstruction is associated with major morbidity; up to 30% of patients suffer loss of kidney function, though renal endometriosis itself is extremely rare.

The symptoms of urinary tract endometriosis are listed in Table 8.2. The diagnosis can be confirmed by:

- ultrasound
- CT and MRI
- cystoscopy
- biopsy – to confirm diagnosis and to exclude malignancy.

In most cases, however, ureteral and renal involvement are diagnosed at the time of open surgical procedure.

The type of treatment chosen should be based on kidney function, the extent and location of the disease, severity of symptoms, age of patient and desire for future pregnancy. If renal function is near normal, hormonal therapy can generally be attempted. Surgery is required for ureteral involvement if there is significant fibrosis and the disease does not respond to hormone treatment.

The recurrence rate of endometriosis in the bladder and ureters is usually very high after medication is stopped, so duration of therapy is important.

Surgery is indicated in cases of acute urinary tract obstruction or when symptoms are severe despite hormonal therapy. The primary surgical treatment of renal endometriosis has been nephrectomy. In patients with bladder endometriosis, partial cystectomy can be performed with good long-term outcome (Figure 8.2).

Thoracic endometriosis

Just over 100 cases of thoracic endometriosis have been reported in the USA and UK. The disease appears to affect women slightly older than those with pelvic endometriosis, the range varying from 15–54 years with an average age of 35 years. Between 50% and 80% of patients have coexisting pelvic endometriosis.

The most common presenting symptom is pneumothorax followed by hemothorax, hemoptysis and asymptomatic lung nodule. Pleural

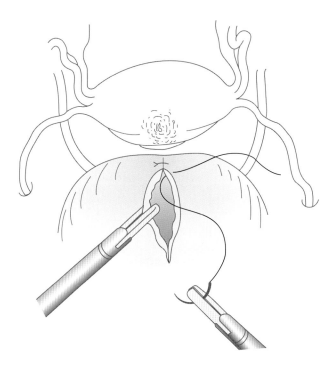

Figure 8.2 Partial cystectomy for the treatment of bladder endometriosis. The bladder is repaired in one layer.

lesions are more likely to cause pneumothorax or hemothorax; hemoptysis is generally the result of lesions in the lung parenchyma.

Total abdominal hysterectomy with bilateral salpingo-oophorectomy has been used in the past as the main form of treatment for extirpation of the origin of thoracic endometriosis. More recently, GnRH agonists and danazol have been used with success in several case reports.

Diaphragmatic endometriosis

Diaphragmatic endometriosis may present as pain in the right upper quadrant or referred pain to the right shoulder. An increasing number of cases have been reported. In one case, a pregnant patient developed hemoperitoneum because of bleeding from an ectopic pregnancy that had implanted on diaphragmatic endometriosis.

Implantation of viable endometrial cells probably occurs following circulation of the cells in a clockwise fashion in the peritoneal fluid. The usual treatment – GnRH agonist and surgery – is reserved for patients with acute symptoms or those who do not respond to other measures. Laparoscopic treatment has also been reported.

Cutaneous endometriosis

Endometriosis involving the skin is limited to the anterior abdominal wall at or below the umbilicus.

Umbilical endometriosis classically presents as a bluish, tender mass, often associated with bleeding. The lesions can be evaluated by ultrasound or radiographically, but the best method is excision biopsy. Treatment is by wide local excision of the disease and the associated scar to reduce the risk of recurrence (reported rate is over 10%).

Inguinal endometriosis presents as a painful mass. Overlying skin changes and cyclic symptoms vary. Endometriosis has been found in hernia sacs, in old inguinal scars and in the inguinal lymphatics. Treatment is by inguinal exploration and excision.

Endometriosis of the nervous system

The most common sites are the nerves in the pelvis. When sciatic pain occurs in relation to the menstrual cycle, it should suggest the presence of endometriosis. Involvement of the obturator nerve may produce pain and weakness in the proximal muscles of the thigh. The treatment is exploration and excision of endometriosis and fibrosis surrounding the nerve.

Endometriosis in men

Endometriosis has been reported in men undergoing treatment for prostate cancer by excision, orchidectomy and high-dose estrogen therapy. The reduction of testosterone after removal of the testicles augmented by estrogen therapy could account for these cases.

Key points – Extrapelvic endometriosis

- Endometriosis occurs outside the pelvis in up to 10% of patients.
- The most common sites for extrapelvic endometriosis are the intestine (especially rectum and sigmoid colon), urinary tract, umbilicus, abdominal wall, lungs, pleura and even the eyes and the nervous system.
- Symptoms of gastrointestinal endometriosis include dyschezia, rectal bleeding, diarrhea and constipation.
- Bladder endometriosis presents as dysuria, frequency of micturition, suprapubic pain and backache.
- Thoracic endometriosis is very rare.
- Cutaneous endometriosis usually occurs at the site of operative scars or the umbilicus.
- Endometriosis may rarely present as inguinal masses.
- Both hormonal therapy and surgery may be used to manage the disease.
- Rarely, endometriosis occurs in men undergoing treatment for prostate cancer by excision, orchidectomy and high-dose estrogen therapy.

Key references

Almedia OD, Val-Gallas JM, Rizk B. Appendectomy under local anesthesia following conscious pain mapping: A report of two cases. *Hum Reprod* 1998;13:588–90.

Chapron C, Boucher E, Fauconnier A et al. Anatomopathological lesions of bladder endometriosis are heterogeneous. *Fertil Steril* 2002;78:740–9.

Jubanyik KJ, Comite F. Extrapelvic endometriosis. Endometriosis. *Obstet Gynecol Clin N Am* 1997;24:411–40.

Nezhat C, Nezhat F, Nezhat C et al. Endometriosis of the intestine and genitourinary tract. In: Nezhat CR, Berger GS, Nezhat FR et al., eds. *Endometriosis: Advanced Management and Surgical Techniques.* New York: Springer, 1995:chapter 15, 137–58.

It has been stated that until we have a technique for identifying all endometriosis in every situation, we have no way of knowing what we are leaving behind at the time of the first surgery; therefore, any endometriosis seen at the second operation may be resistant rather than recurrent. This is true for superficial, peritoneal endometriosis, as the lesions might have been microscopic, and also true for deep endometriosis, which could have been retroperitoneal and concealed. Even with good medical and surgical management, endometriosis is a progressive disease that tends to recur after treatment. The reasons for recurrent/persistent endometriosis are:

- evolution of lesions
- persistence of the disease due to deficient recognition of visible but subtle lesions
- imperfect identification of subperitoneal lesions
- incomplete excision at laparoscopy or laparotomy
- uterosacral endometriosis not excised at the time of hysterectomy.

The diagnosis of recurrence is based on the symptoms and signs, and physical examination, together with transvaginal ultrasonography, MRI or CA-125 immunoassay if appropriate.

Recurrence rate after laparotomy. In 1953, Meigs noted the recurrence of symptoms in 7% (15/215) of patients, but did not reoperate on any patient. Punnonen, in the largest study published, observed a recurrence rate of 15% in a 6–10 year follow-up of 903 patients surgically treated for the disease. Wheeler and Malinak, in a classic study of 423 patients, documented a 10% recurrence rate; the annual recurrence rate varied from 1% (first year) to 14% in the eighth year, with a cumulative rate of 14% at 3 years and 40% at 5 years.

Recurrence after laparoscopic surgery. Fayez and colleagues reported on 162 women with infertility and stage I or II endometriosis: 82 had laparoscopic excision and 80 took danazol, 600 mg/day, for 6 months.

Follow-up laparoscopy 1 year later confirmed that the disease had recurred in 4% (3/28) and 9% (7/19) of the two groups, respectively.

Redwine and colleagues demonstrated a 5-year cumulative recurrence rate of 10% among 359 women with endometriosis (stages I–IV), who were treated by laparoscopic excision and followed up for 2 years. Canis and colleagues found 10% of patients had persistent lesions after excision of deep ovarian endometriomas.

Recurrence after medical treatment. Evers and colleagues found the recurrence rate after medical therapy to be 29–51%. The difference between various recurrence rates is due to the length of time before follow-up, and diagnosis of recurrence (by the patient's symptoms or by laparoscopy, with or without histological confirmation). Evers advised against second-look laparoscopy during medical therapy. Shaw and colleagues estimated recurrence at 36% in early endometriosis, increasing to 76% in patients with advanced endometriosis.

Recurrence after hysterectomy with and without bilateral salpingo-oophorectomy. Recurrence of symptoms and reoperation rate after total abdominal hysterectomy with and without bilateral salpingo-oophorectomy is presented in Table 9.1. As previously stated, Horowitz and colleagues suggested that recurrent pain following hysterectomy may be due to persistent endometriosis in uterosacral ligaments. They recommended surgical excision for these patients.

Hormone replacement therapy. The relationship between recurrent endometriosis and hormone replacement therapy (HRT) is complicated and needs further research. Every patient should be fully counselled and her management individualized.

After radical surgery, the incidence of recurrence of the disease is thought to be rare. In 1970, Ranney reported no recurrences when estrogen replacement was not given, and 3% when it was. In 1973, Gray reported no recurrences when no hormones were given and 20% when they were. Importantly, most recurrences included bowel involvement with endometriosis.

TABLE 9.1

Recurrence of symptoms and reoperations after total abdominal hysterectomy with or without bilateral salpingo-oophorectomy

Author	Year	Recurrence of symptoms (%)	Reoperations (%)
TAH without BSO			
Sheets et al., Ranney	1963, 1970	–	1–3
Andrews & Larsen	1976	–	85
Hammond et al.	1976	–	85
Wilson	1988	3	–
Walters	1989	7	–
Henderson & Studd	1991	–	25
Namnoum et al.	1995	62	31
TAH with BSO			
Henderson & Studd	1991	–	1.1
Walters	1988	8	–
Namnoum et al.	1995	10	3.7

TAH, total abdominal hysterectomy; BSO, bilateral salpingo-oophorectomy

In a retrospective cohort study, Hickman et al. treated patients with estrogen replacement therapy (ERT) after total abdominal hysterectomy and bilateral salpingo-oophorectomy. The timing of initiated ERT was correlated with success in 60 women who began ERT in the immediate postoperative period. Of these, 4 (7%) had recurrent pain, whereas 7 (20%) of 35 women who began ERT more than 6 weeks postoperatively experienced recurrent pain. This was not statistically significant; it seems the early start of ERT did not affect the recurrence of pain. When controlled for length of patient follow-up and adjusted for stage, age and postoperative hydroxyprogesterone therapy, the results showed that those who started ERT more than 6 weeks postoperatively had a relative risk of 5.7 (95% CI 1.3–25.2) for pain recurrence.

Recurrent ovarian endometrioma is a common problem. The incidence depends on the technique and varies from 8% to 22%. Obviously, the more aggressive the ultrasonographic follow-up, the higher the chance of identifying recurrent endometriomas. Early recurrences may be related to inadequate surgical procedure. Two possibilities exist: inadequate treatment of the cyst or missing a second or third endometrioma. These problems are more common in patients with extensive adhesions.

In young patients, it is better to plan to treat recurrent ovarian endometrioma than to induce menopause by surgery. In older patients, an aggressive approach and even oophorectomy may be used. Microsurgical techniques should be performed with adequate hemostasis and great care to avoid damage to the ovary. In desperate cases where repeat laparoscopies and laparotomies have been performed, transvaginal aspiration may be an option, despite the high recurrence rate.

Recurrent deep endometriosis. Koninckx reviewed the Leuven database of 2482 women with endometriosis and found that the recurrence rate for deep endometriosis is extremely low. In these cases, the endometriosis was probably missed at the first laparoscopy or was incompletely removed.

Prevention of recurrent endometriosis by postoperative medical therapy. Randomized, double-blind, controlled trials have demonstrated the efficacy of laparoscopic endometriosis ablation in increasing the pregnancy rate in infertile women and in reducing pelvic pain in symptomatic patients. The question we now pose is: what impact does postoperative medical therapy have on the recurrence of endometriosis? Vercellini and colleagues recently reviewed randomized and non-randomized controlled clinical studies published in the last decades in the English language to determine the impact of postoperative medical therapy on recurrence, pain and fertility. Three randomized controlled trials and one retrospective cohort study fulfilled all the criteria for review. The results do not support the notion that suppressing ovarian activity postoperatively increases the long term pregnancy rate, which is similar to previous meta-analyses. As far as pelvic pain is concerned, more data was needed, as one randomized trial suggested a decrease in symptoms and recurrence while another did not. The authors analyzed their own case series and could not demonstrate any protective effect of postoperative medical therapy on the incidence of recurrence after conservative surgery.

Usual causes of recurrence

Ovarian remnant syndrome occurs if the ovary is not completely removed at the time of the surgery, possibly because of dense pelvic adhesions to the pelvic side-wall, or to the bladder and ureters. The most common presentation of this syndrome is pain unrelieved by analgesics. Measurement of FSH is useful in making the diagnosis, but this also relies on histological confirmation of ovarian tissue obtained at the time of the operation.

Steroid receptors and endometriosis. Metzger and colleagues have demonstrated that the hormonal responsiveness of endometrial implants is inconsistent, possibly as a result of faulty regulation of steroid hormone receptors.

Extrapelvic endometriosis in postmenopausal women has been reported in several cases, who may or may not have had endometriosis at an earlier age. The most common sites for the disease were the urinary tract and bowel.

Management of recurrent endometriosis

The methods of treating recurrent endometriosis are outlined in Figure 9.1.

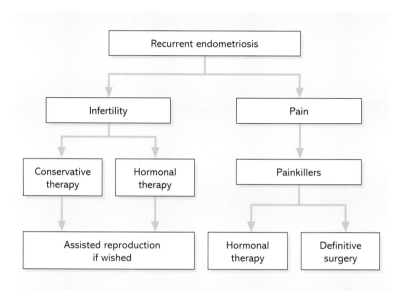

Figure 9.1 Treatment options for recurrent endometriosis.

Key points – Recurrent endometriosis

- Recurrence may be due to evolution, persistence or incomplete excision of the lesions.
- The recurrence rate following laparotomy is 10% after 12 months, 14% after 3 years and 40% after 5 years.
- The recurrence rate of endometriosis after conservative laparoscopic surgery is 4–10% after 12 months.
- The recurrence rate of endometriosis after medical therapy is high (29–51%).
- Postoperative medical therapy may prolong the time before recurrence.
- The recurrence rate of ovarian endometriomas is 8–22%. In young women, it is better to deal with recurrence than to induce surgical menopause.
- Recurrence after hysterectomy is likely to be due to residual disease in the uterosacral ligaments.

Key references

Aboulghar MA, Mansour RT, Rizk B et al. Ultrasonic transvaginal aspiration of endometriotic cysts: an optional line of treatment in selected cases of endometriosis. *Hum Reprod* 1991;6:1408–10.

Candiani GB, Fedele L, Bianchi S. Recurrent endometriosis. In: Nezhat CR, Berger GS, Nezhat FR et al., eds. *Endometriosis: Advanced Management and Surgical Techniques.* New York: Springer, 1995:chapter 16, 159–71.

Canis M, Botchorishvili R, Schindler L et al. Recurrent ovarian endometrioma. In: Lemay A, Maheux R, eds. *Understanding and Managing Endometriosis: Advances in Research and Practice.* New York: Parthenon, 1999:chapter 37, 245–50.

Hasty LA, Murphy AA. Management of recurrent endometriosis after hysterectomy and bilateral salpingo-oophorectomy. In: Nezhat CR, Berger GS, Nezhat FR et al., eds. *Endometriosis: Advanced Management and Surgical Techniques.* New York: Springer, 1995:chapter 18, 189–92.

Koninckx PR. Recurrence rate of deep endometriosis. In: Lemay A, Maheux R, eds. *Understanding and Managing Endometriosis: Advances in Research and Practice.* New York: Parthenon, 1999:chapter 38, 251–59.

Meigs JV. Endometriosis – etiologic role of marriage and parity; conservative treatment. *Obstet Gynecol* 1953;2:46–53.

Vercellini P, De Giorgio O, Pesole A et al. Prevention of recurrences by postoperative medical treatment. In: Lemay A, Maheux R, eds. *Understanding and Managing Endometriosis: Advances in Research and Practice.* New York: Parthenon, 1999:chapter 39, 261–8.

Adenomyosis is the invasion of the myometrium by the endometrial glands and/or stroma. The complaint is more common in women who have had children than those who have not, and generally appears between the ages of 40 to 70 years. It was first described in 1860 by Rokitansky, who noted a condition in which endometrial glands in hyperplastic muscular stroma invaded the uterine wall; the nature of the growth of these areas suggested sarcomatoid changes. In 1896, Cullen suggested the term 'adenomyosis' and subsequently published a review of 54 cases of what would be recognized today as adenomyosis.

Though often called endometriosis interna, adenomyosis is present simultaneously with endometriosis in fewer than one in four patients. The glands appear histologically similar to the basalis part of the endometrium, so they do not usually undergo the proliferative and secretory changes associated with cyclic ovarian hormone production. The diagnosis rests on finding these glands beneath the endometrial surface, within the uterine muscle layer.

Prevalence

Published material gives a widely varying prevalence rate. Adenomyosis is usually diagnosed incidentally by the pathologist examining surgical specimens, so prevalence relates directly to such research. More than 60% of women in the 40–70-year age range may be affected.

Pathogenesis

Guarnaccia described how, over the years, four primary theories have been proposed to explain adenomyosis: heredity, trauma, hyperestrogenemia and viral transmission. The accepted hypothesis is that high estrogen levels stimulate hyperplasia of the basalis layer of the endometrium, thus causing the barrier between the endometrium and myometrium to break down. The stroma and subsequently the glands begin to invade the myometrium along the path of least resistance; in most cases, this growth is adjacent to lymphatic and vascular channels.

The reason for the occurrence of this downgrowth could be a mechanical factor, such as childbirth or curettage. Chronic inflammation could also damage the endometrial and myometrial borders and facilitate endometrial downgrowth.

Estrogen receptors are always found in adenomyomatous tissue, though in reduced quantity compared with normal myometrium. If progesterone receptors are present, they are found in fewer numbers than in normal endometrium.

Pathology

The two forms of adenomyosis are:

- distinct
- diffuse (more common).

Both the anterior and posterior walls of the uterus can be involved, though the disease is more likely to occur in the posterior wall. In the diffuse form, there are no encapsulated areas of adenomyosis. The uterus is enlarged asymmetrically up to three times its normal size (about the size it would be at 14 weeks' gestation). The cut surface has a spongy appearance and protrudes convexly (Figure 10.1).

The standard criterion for diagnosis is the presence of endometrial glands and stroma 3 mm or more from the basalis layer of the endometrium. Histologically, the glands exhibit an inactive or proliferative pattern.

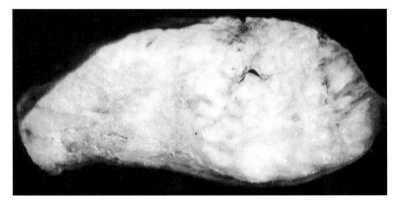

Figure 10.1 Cut surface of a uterus showing diffuse and distinct adenomyosis. Reproduced with permission from Nezhat CR et al. 1995.

Associated gynecologic pathology. Adenomyosis rarely occurs as an isolated finding. Up to 80% of adenomyotic uteri are associated with such conditions as leiomyomata, endometrial hyperplasia, peritoneal endometriosis and uterine cancer (Table 10.1). Endometrial hyperplasia is common. In rare cases where adenocarcinoma develops, the diagnosis can be extremely difficult. Symptoms are lacking and there is no diagnostic tool other than hysterectomy; Woodruff et al. have, however, found malignant cells in cervical smears from such patients. There have also been various reports of a high prevalence of adenomyosis in patients with endometrial cancer, but there are no data to suggest that adenomyosis predisposes to malignant degeneration.

Clinical diagnosis

The most frequently cited profile of adenomyosis symptomatology includes the triad of abnormal uterine bleeding, secondary dysmenorrhea and enlarged uterus. Other symptoms such as dyspareunia and pelvic pain present less commonly (Table 10.2). However, none of those symptoms are pathognomonic for adenomyosis. Because adenomyosis is frequently accompanied by other pelvic pathology (Table 10.1), it is often difficult to attribute symptoms solely to this condition. Furthermore, up to 35% of affected patients may be asymptomatic.

TABLE 10.1

Association of adenomyosis with other gynecologic pathology

Condition	Reported association (%)
Uterine leiomyomata	19–57
Endometrial hyperplasia	7–33
Endometriosis	0–28
Salpingitis isthmica nodosa	1–20

Data from Guarnaccia MM, Silverberg K, Olive DL. Endometriosis and adenomyosis. In: Copeland LJ, ed. *Textbook of Gynecology*, 2nd edn. Philadelphia, WB Saunders, 1999.

TABLE 10.2

Adenomyosis symptomatology

Symptom	Reported incidence (%)
Menorrhagia	51–68
Metrorrhagia	11–39
Dysmenorrhea	20–46
Dyspareunia	7
Asymptomatic	3–35

Data from Guarnaccia MM, Silverberg K, Olive DL. Endometriosis and adenomyosis. In: Copeland LJ, ed. *Textbook of Gynecology*, 2nd edn. Philadelphia, WB Saunders, 1999.

Investigations

Myometrial biopsy remains the gold standard for a diagnosis without a hysterectomy specimen (Figure 10.2). These biopsies can be obtained by means of laparotomy, laparoscopy or hysteroscopy, and techniques are continually improving. Unfortunately, many cases can be overlooked unless the disease is extensive. McCausland used a 27 Fr operative hysteroscope and took biopsies of the posterior wall with a 5 mm loop electrode in 90 patients. This study confirmed the efficacy of the procedure, with no complications of either bleeding or perforation. However, this technique is contraindicated in postmenopausal women, because of the high risk of perforating the thin uterine wall.

Ultrasound. Both transabdominal and transvaginal ultrasound have been used to diagnose adenomyosis, with a positive predictive value of 70%.

MRI is the ideal procedure. In expert hands, it is most sensitive and can differentiate between adenomyosis and the presence of fibroids.

Hysteroscopy. On rare occasions, visualization of a small endometrial diverticulum during hysteroscopy can raise suspicion of adenomyosis.

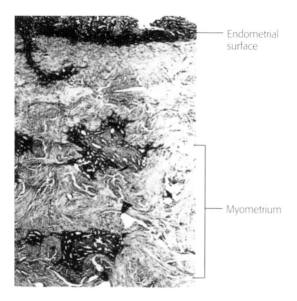

Endometrial surface

Myometrium

Figure 10.2 Myometrial biopsy showing islands of endometrial tissue deep within the myometrium. Reproduced with permission from Janovski NA et al. *Atlas of Gynecological and Obstetric Diagnostic Histopathology.* New York: McGraw-Hill 1967.

Hysterosalpingography is poor in confirming or excluding a diagnosis of adenomyosis.

CA-125. Data from a study comparing levels of the ovarian epithelial tumor antigen CA-125 in patients with adenomyosis and in patients with fibroids were contradictory. However, if ectopic endometrium produces CA-125, the serum levels in patients with adenomyosis should be higher and therapy should lower the CA-125 concentration. It is hoped further investigation in this area will be encouraging.

Treatment of adenomyosis

Hysterectomy is the definitive treatment if the patient's age and parity permit. Preoperative endometrial sampling should be carried out to exclude malignancy. The route of hysterectomy (abdominal or vaginal) and whether bilateral oophorectomy is required is determined by age and other surgical conditions.

Endomyometrial resection. Through advances in diagnostic imaging, conservative intervention such as endomyometrial ablation or endomyometrial resection have been proposed. Simple endometrial ablation is not able to resolve adenomyosis because, by definition, this is too deep. Ablation must go much deeper, or endomyometrial resection or myometrial excision has to be performed. Conservative surgery using endomyometrial ablation, laparoscopic myometrial electrocoagulation, or excision of adenomyosis has been helpful in some patients, although so far follow-up is restricted to 3 years.

Levonorgestrel-releasing IUD. Menorrhagia associated with adenomyosis has recently been successfully treated with an IUD that releases levonorgestrel, 20 µg/day; it is inserted within 7 days of menstruation.

Danazol-releasing IUD. In a study from 1993–2000, women with adenomyotic uteri were treated with IUDs containing danazol; dysmenorrhea and CA-125 levels decreased significantly. In patients with endometrial hyperplasia, the hyperplasia disappeared after danazol treatment.

Medical treatment of adenomyosis consists of GnRH agonists, danazol, cyclic hormones and prostaglandin synthetase inhibitors for pain and abnormal uterine bleeding. Two patients receiving GnRH therapy carried a pregnancy to full term.

A recent study examined the effects of a novel, orally active matrix metalloproteinase inhibitor, ONO-4817, on uterine adenomyosis induced in mice by pituitary grafting. The results indicate that ONO-4817 may be an effective inhibitor of the development of adenomyosis.

Adenomyosis in pregnancy

A large study of 151 uteri obtained at Cesarean hysterectomy found an incidence of adenomyosis of 17.2%. Although fifty years ago it was suggested that adenomyosis in pregnancy markedly increases uterine atony and rupture, this has not proven to be the case. Azziz noted only

29 cases of complications in more than eighty years of literature, a surprisingly low figure in light of the incidence of adenomyosis of pregnancy.

Key points – Adenomyosis

- Adenomyosis is the invasion of myometrium by endometrial glands and stroma.
- Uterine leiomyoma, endometrial hyperplasia, salpingitis isthmica nodosa and endometrial carcinoma are frequently associated pathologies.
- The most common symptoms are menorrhagia, metrorrhagia, dysmenorrhea and dyspareunia.
- Many patients with adenomyosis are asymptomatic.
- Hysterectomy is the definitive treatment for adenomyosis.
- Gonadotropin-releasing hormone agonists are the medical treatment of choice; levonorgestrel intrauterine devices and danazol intrauterine devices are other options.
- Matrix metalloproteinase inhibitors have been used successfully in animal studies.

Key references

Azziz R. Adenomyosis in pregnancy: a review. *J Reprod Med* 1986;31:224.

Azziz R. Adenomyosis: current perspectives. *Obstet Gynecol Clin N Am* 1989;16:221–35.

Brosens JJ, Brosens I. Endometriosis and adenomyosis: a unifying hypothesis. In: Lemay A, Maheux R, eds. *Understanding and Managing Endometriosis: Advances in Research and Practice*. New York: Parthenon, 1999:chapter 3, 11–16.

Droegemueller W. Endometriosis and adenomyosis. In: Mishell DR, Stenchever MA, Droegemueller W et al., eds. *Comprehensive gynecology*. St Louis: Mosby, 1997:18.

Jen SW, Lim-Tan SK, Wee D et al. The clinical significance of adenomyosis and its relation to fertility. In *Advances in fertility and sterility series*, vol 5. London: Parthenon, 1987:207–12.

Mori T, Yamasaki S, Masui F et al. Suppression of the development of experimentally induced uterine adenomyosis by a novel matrix metalloproteinase inhibitor, ONO-4817, in mice. *Exp Biol Med* 2001;226:429–33.

In the many thousands of papers published about the disease there have been many references to the puzzle that is endometriosis. For those with the disease, the fact that it is 'a riddle wrapped in a mystery inside an enigma' (as one specialist wrote) will not bring comfort. Their hope is that a solution will be found that will eradicate the pain and suffering they endure while the disease is present.

Because of its nature, a diagnosis of endometriosis (Table 11.1) will be the start of a long-term, ongoing relationship with a family practitioner and gynecologist. It is important that the professionals establish this at the earliest stage, showing interest and concern in the person and her general well-being. You have to take trouble to communicate, to obtain the essential facts, and explain both the illness and the treatment options in a way that she understands, so that she can appreciate the choices open to her. Encourage questions and suggest ways she can find out more about her condition through reading or self-help groups.

TABLE 11.1

The family practitioner's checklist for investigating endometriosis

- Take a comprehensive history, asking about start of menarche, physical reactions to menstruation such as pain before, after or during, regularity and duration of menstruation

- Check out the risk factors (see Table 1.1)

- Ask about other pain that may be relevant to the diagnosis; remind yourself that pain can have psychological consequences, and that a patient showing despair in conjunction with other symptoms might be a victim of this progressive disease

- During the physical examination note specific and non-specific findings and check them out (see Tables 3.1, 3.2, 3.3)

- Arrange for further tests or refer the person directly to a specialist

She will want to know about pain and discomfort she might experience (over and above that of the disease itself), the risks of the proposed treatments, including anything that might affect her ability to have a child, the side effects, how much time is involved in treatment, whether she will need to take time off work, whether she will be incapacitated and need help with her family.

If she asks about a second opinion, encourage her with the name of another specialist in endometriosis. She needs to be reassured that treatment suggested is appropriate. This is especially important if she has been told she must have a hysterectomy, or if nothing further can be done to treat the disease.

Where conventional treatment is not successful, it may in some cases be useful to suggest coping strategies to deal with the primary symptom of pain: gentle heat applied to the abdomen or lower back, non-jarring exercise such as swimming and walking, acupuncture, physiotherapy, reflexology, use of relaxation and visualization tapes. Encourage her to help herself, to enter into a partnership of treatment.

Useful addresses

The National Endometriosis Society
Suite 50, Westminster Palace Gardens
1–7 Artillery Row
London SW1P 1RL UK
Tel: 020 7222 2781 (administration)
(freephone UK) 0808 808 2227 (national helpline 14.00–17.00
Mondays and Tuesdays, 19.00–22.00 daily)
Fax: 020 7222 2786
www.endo.org.uk

Simply Holistic Endometriosis (SHE) Trust
14 Moorland Way
Lincoln LN6 7JW UK
Tel/Fax: 0870 7743665/4
shetrust@shetrust.org.uk
www.shetrust.org.uk
The SHE Trust focuses on alternative treatments for
endometriosis as well as conventional treatments

Endometriosis Association International Headquarters
8585 North 76th Place
Milwaukee WI 53223 USA
Tel: 414 355 2200
(toll-free N America and Caribbean) 1 800 992 3636
Fax: 414 355 6065
endo@EndometriosisAssn.org
www.endometriosisassn.org

Index